THE SUPER-CHARGED
HORMONE DIET

A **30-DAY** Accelerated Plan
to Lose Weight,
Restore Metabolism
& **Feel Younger Longer**

DR. NATASHA TURNER
Naturopathic Doctor
Author of *The Hormone Diet* and
The Carb Sensitivity Program

RODALE.

Mention of specific companies, organizations, or authorities in this book
does not imply endorsement by the author or publisher, nor does mention
of specific companies, organizations, or authorities imply that they
endorse this book, its author, or the publisher.

Internet addresses and telephone numbers given in this book were accurate at the time
it went to press.

First published in Canada by Random House Canada in 2011.

© 2011 by Essence Wellness Inc.

This edition is being reprinted in November 2013 by Rodale Inc.
with permission from Random House Canada.

Rodale books may be purchased for business or promotional use or for special sales.
For information, please write to:

Special Markets Department, Rodale Inc., 733 Third Avenue, New York, NY 10017

Printed in the United States of America
Rodale Inc. makes every effort to use acid-free ♾, recycled paper ♲.

Text design by Terri Nimo

Library of Congress Cataloging-in-Publication Data is on file with the publisher.

ISBN 978–1–62336–289–8   hardcover

Distributed to the trade by Macmillan

2   4   6   8   10   9   7   5   3   1   hardcover

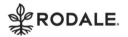

We inspire and enable people to improve their lives and the world around them.
rodalebooks.com

For Timmy,
We've grown up together and
we're still growing . . .

CONTENTS

PART ONE

The secret of getting ahead is getting started.

MARK TWAIN

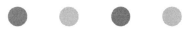

CHAPTER 1

OUR BIG FAT
HORMONAL IMBALANCES

*Insanity: doing the same thing over and over again
and expecting different results.*

ALBERT EINSTEIN

Imagine exercising daily, counting calories and excluding food groups only to have your belly fat or love handles grow bigger and bigger. The more you strive to meet your goal, the further you are from achieving it. It's the always shocking, incredibly frustrating, unsuccessful dieting phenomenon. And it happened to me.

At the time, I was a student and I assumed that the diet and exercise program I was following wasn't strict enough, long enough, or strenuous enough. Naturally I decided that I simply needed to do them both—harder. So, in desperation I added more cardio sessions and further reduced my food intake. The result? I gained another 5 pounds on top of the 20 I had already piled on. How could this be?

Let's recall my equation for fat loss from *The Hormone Diet*:

Lasting fat loss = hormonal balance + (calories in − calories burned)

My intense efforts failed because they only served to make my hormonal imbalance, the true underlying cause of my weight gain, *worse*. Unbeknownst to me, I had a deficiency of thyroid hormone going on in the background. The imbalance only grew worse because the physical stress associated with excessive caloric restriction and over-exercising actually *increased* the negative impact on my thyroid hormone deficiency and *further* slowed my metabolism. After this, three things quickly became very clear to me. First, weight loss is by no means only about calories in versus calories out—hormonal balance needed to be added to the equation. Second, hormones are very powerful substances that influence many aspects of our health and well-being. And third, the level of one hormone impacts another, which established the need to think "big picture" when it comes to weight loss.

So, if we now know this as the new formula for fat loss, then surely we need to start thinking about *all* the factors that upset our hormonal balance and, therefore, ultimately make us fat. But I'll tell you a secret before we get into a discussion of the eight most common fat-packing hormonal imbalances and the reasons why we are fat. This program fixes them all.

Tackling the Taboo Topic of Hormonal Health

After the release of my first book, *The Hormone Diet,* I received hundreds of emails from people around the globe expressing exuberant relief that they finally found some answers. Many felt as if the book had been written directly for them, and they had at last discovered a solution to their nagging symptoms and hormonal hurdles. People were no longer sweeping their issues under the carpet, making excuses or hitting a wall with no discernible answers. It was exactly why I wrote the book in the first place—to create **a practical guidebook that explains the cause, the effect and the solution, so people can make informed decisions about their own health—one step at a time.** But a lot of readers also requested my three-step wellness plan to be more simply laid out. They wanted a more direct pathway to successful solutions—without the science. And so herein lies *The Supercharged Hormone Diet* 30-Day plan. I want better health to be accessible to everyone, and this plan is so clear anyone can do it.

The pace of life just seems to get more and more hectic. Between work, family and other obligations, we're all finding ourselves stretched—and stressed. Unfortunately, this busy lifestyle often leads us to place our health at the bottom of the priority list. Without realizing it, we find ourselves beholden to a host of poor habits—eating on the run, skipping workouts, grabbing too few hours of sleep and dismissing everyday symptoms that are often red flags for something more serious. These habits leave us carrying excess pounds, looking drained and feeling just plain bad. Often we respond by seeking a quick fix to lose weight. But when our bodies are so out of balance, long-term weight loss is next to impossible. This book is about *all* the aspects of your lifestyle that come together to make—or break—your weight-loss success. It's about taking the time and some simple steps to make yourself, your health and your overall well-being a top priority again.

Think about what drew you to this book in the first place. Do you have trouble dragging yourself out of bed in the morning? Do you experience uncontrollable sugar cravings at 3 p.m.? Nagging PMS every month? Interrupted sleep patterns? Do you get stressed out just sitting in your office? Do you have difficulty coping with every task? Bloating after meals? Skin that has lost its luster or tone? Belly fat that just won't go away? The list can go on and on, and I am willing to bet that many of you experience some of these frustrations every day. Believe it or not, these aren't just factors that make you feel bad. They are impacting your ability to lose weight!

Unfortunately, many of us are too embarrassed or too used to the symptoms to even think about discussing or addressing them. Both women and men have spent too long believing that their hormonal symptoms are a liability or are psychosomatic to simply be ignored. Yet hormones are powerful chemical messengers in our body—they control everything from our reproductive functions to our mood, sleep, appearance and almost every other aspect of daily life. The very same hormones that are behind a whole host of health concerns (such as the ones listed above) are also influencing your ability to control your appetite, shed body fat and gain lean muscle. They dictate how successful we will be with a given weight-loss program; whether we will be able to drop unwanted pounds or continue on the diet merry-go-round to no avail. So many of us believe we can get healthy by losing weight. But it was my goal to teach you in *The Hormone Diet* that *we must be healthy in order to lose weight.*

The Eight Most Common Fat-Packing Hormonal Imbalances

If you have been unable to lose weight, even with diet and exercise, your hormones are very likely the reason you have not been successful. Our bodies are hard-wired to send us signals when something isn't right, but often we're too busy to hear them begging for attention. Many of us experience signs and symptoms of hormonal imbalance every day. Recognizing and treating the subtle signs of hormonal imbalance is essential, yet so many of us have been out of balance for so many years that we don't know how to recognize what "balance" is anymore.

No matter how an imbalance manifests on the outside, the internal reality remains the same—*any and all hormonal imbalance leads to difficulty losing weight and increased risk of obesity.* Unfortunately, the most common imbalances cannot be solved by dieting alone. In fact, they can *prevent successful fat loss,* even when great diet and exercise plans are in place. If you have not been successful in the past, one or more of the following hormonal imbalances could be the culprit:

Inflammation: Digestive disorders, allergies, autoimmune disease, arthritis, asthma, eczema, acne, abdominal fat, headaches, depression and sinus disorders are all associated with chronic inflammation, which has recently become recognized as the root cause of obesity and unhealthy aging. At the 2007 Postgraduate Nutrition Symposium at Harvard University, researchers revealed findings suggesting that inflammation and excess insulin are *the* major contributors to rising rates of type 2 diabetes and the overall fattening of North America.

Insulin Excess: Insulin is an essential substance whose main function is to process sugar in the bloodstream and carry it into cells to be used as fuel or stored as fat. There are several reasons for excess insulin, but the main culprits are stress, consuming too much nutrient-poor carbohydrate (the type found in processed foods, sugary drinks and sodas, packaged low-fat foods and artificial sweeteners) insufficient protein intake, inadequate fat intake and deficient fiber consumption. Heart palpitations, sweating, poor concentration, weakness, anxiety, fogginess, fatigue, irritability or impaired thinking are common short-term side effects of high insulin. Unfortunately, our body typically responds to these unpleasant feelings by making us think we're hungry, which in turn causes us to reach for more high-sugar foods and drinks. We then end up in a vicious cycle of hormonal imbalance, a condition called insulin resistance or metabolic syndrome, which only furthers weight gain and our risk of diabetes and heart disease.

Depression or Anxiety: Serotonin exerts powerful influence over mood, emotions, memory, cravings (especially for carbohydrates), self-esteem, pain tolerance, sleep habits, appetite, digestion and body temperature regulation. When we're feeling down or depressed, we naturally crave more sugars and starches to stimulate the production of serotonin. The World Health Organization (WHO) projects that depression and anxiety will soon be the number-one disability experienced by adults. For adequate serotonin production, all of the following are crucial: plenty of sunlight; a healthy diet rich in protein, minerals and vitamins; regular exercise and good sleep. When we measure our current lifestyle against all the elements necessary for the body's natural production of serotonin, the wide-ranging epidemic of low serotonin is certainly not surprising. Add in chronic stress and out-of-control multitasking—two of the main causes of serotonin depletion—and it's no wonder many of us suffer from depleted serotonin.

Chronic Stress: Under situations of chronic stress—whether the stress is physical, emotional, mental, environmental, *real or imagined*—our body releases high amounts of the hormone cortisol. If you suffer from a mood disorder such as anxiety, depression, post-traumatic stress disorder or exhaustion, or if you have a digestive issue such as irritable bowel syndrome, you can bet your body is cranking up your cortisol. Through a complicated network of hormonal interactions, prolonged stress results in a raging appetite, metabolic decline, belly fat and a loss of hard-won, metabolically active muscle tissue. In other words, chronic stress makes us soft, flabby and much older than we truly are!

Toxic Estrogen: Researchers have now identified excess estrogen to be *as great a risk factor for obesity*—in both sexes—as poor eating habits and lack of exercise. There are two ways to accumulate excess estrogen in the body: we either produce too much of it on our own or acquire it from our environment or diet. We are constantly exposed to estrogen-like compounds in foods that contain toxic pesticides, herbicides and growth hormones. A premenopausal woman with estrogen dominance will likely have PMS, too much body fat around the hips and difficulty losing weight. Menopausal women and, yes, men too, may experience low libido, memory loss, poor motivation, depression, loss of muscle mass and increased belly fat.

Menopause: According to projections by consumer reports in the Unites States, 25 million women will hit menopause within the next decade. Contrary to popular belief, menopause, which can begin as early as 40 years of age, is not just about estrogen decline. Supplies of other hormones such as progesterone, testosterone and dehydroepiandrosterone (DHEA) also tend to dry up, right along with the skin, hair, eyes and libido. So many women come to my office intensely frustrated with the unwelcome changes in their body during this phase of life, especially an annoying thickening of the waistline. Other common symptoms of menopause include hot flashes, difficulty sleeping, headaches, heart palpitations, poor memory and concentration, urinary urgency or incontinence, vaginal dryness, changes in the appearance of skin and hair and emotional changes including depression, anxiety and irritability.

Low Testosterone: Testosterone enhances libido, bone density, muscle mass, strength, motivation, memory, fat burning and skin tone in both men and women. An increase of body fat and loss of muscle may happen, even with dieting and exercise, when testosterone is low. Testosterone levels tend to taper off with aging, obesity and stress, but today men are experiencing testosterone decline much earlier in life. This is quite an alarming finding, considering low testosterone has been linked to depression, obesity, osteoporosis, heart disease *and even death.* Dr. Mitchell Harman, an endocrinologist at the University of Arizona College of Medicine, blames the proliferation of endocrine-suppressing estrogen-like compounds used in pesticides and other farming chemicals for the downward trend in male testosterone levels. Phthalates, commonly found in cosmetics, soaps and most plastics, are another known cause of testosterone suppression.

Hypothyroidism: Without enough thyroid hormone, every system in the body slows down. Those who suffer from hypothyroidism feel tired, tend to sleep a lot, experience constipation and typically experience weight gain. Extremely dry skin, hair loss, slower mental processes, brittle hair, splitting nails, diminished ability to sweat during exercise, infertility, poor memory, depression, decreased libido, feeling cold or an inability to lose weight are also symptoms to watch for. If you suspect you have a thyroid condition, make sure your doctor assesses you and your full range of symptoms, *not just your blood work.* Even levels of TSH (an indicator of thyroid function) within the normal range have been proven to accelerate weight gain and to interfere with a healthy metabolic rate in both men and women.

If you don't know whether your hormones are in balance or not, or if you may be experiencing one of the eight most common fat-packing hormonal imbalances, don't worry; you will be able to assess whether one or more imbalances are influencing your health by taking my Hormonal Health Profile in Chapter 11.

Since hormones control our appetite and stimulate metabolism, achieving and maintaining hormonal balance plays an *essential* role in achieving lasting fat loss. Yes, diet and exercise are important. But the lasting solution must also include sleeping well, conquering inflammation, detoxification, optimizing digestion, limiting stress and introducing supplements or natural (bio-identical) hormone replacement. All of these factors influence our hormonal activity—and, ultimately, our weight-loss success—in truly dramatic ways.

YOUR FAT-LOSS FOES			
THE HORMONES AND CONDITIONS THAT INTERFERE WITH FAT BURNING, BOOST APPETITE AND CAUSE WEIGHT GAIN			
FAT-LOSS FOE	THE PERFECT BALANCE	THE IMBALANCE THAT CAUSES FAT GAIN	*THE SUPERCHARGED HORMONE DIET* RECOMMENDATION THAT HELPS RESTORE BALANCE
Insulin, the hormone that regulates blood sugar. It is the ONLY hormone that is always telling your body to store energy as fat. See page 7 for more information on insulin excess.	Not too high, not too low.	Excess insulin (Insulin Resistance or Metabolic Syndrome) usually arising as a result of poor diet, lack of exercise, excess alcohol consumption, stress or sleep deprivation.	Great sleep and stress management; detoxification; hormonally balanced nutrition and supplements; exercise (particularly strength training); additional recommendations in Chapter 11, pages 190–93 if you need targeted help for excess insulin.

FAT-LOSS FOE	THE PERFECT BALANCE	THE IMBALANCE THAT CAUSES FAT GAIN	THE SUPERCHARGED HORMONE DIET RECOMMENDATION THAT HELPS RESTORE BALANCE
Estrogen, the sex hormone dominant in the first half of the menstrual cycle. Excess estrogen is a major cause of weight gain for both men and women. For more information see page 8, section on toxic excess estrogen.	Not too high, not too low.	Excess estrogen (Estrogen Dominance), which usually arises from estrogen exposure in our environment or because we fail to eliminate estrogen via regular bowel movements and liver detoxification.	Great sleep and stress management; detoxification, especially with the help of the Clear Detox—Hormonal Health (Clear Medicine); hormonally balanced nutrition and supplements; exercise; additional recommendations in Chapter 11, pages 203–5 if you need targeted help for this specific hormone.
Ghrelin, the hormone released from the stomach that increases appetite.	Not too high.	Excess ghrelin released as a result of sleep deprivation or in between meals to trigger hunger (when your stomach is growling!)	Great sleep and stress management; good nutrition.
Inflammation Not a hormone but a definite cause of hormonal imbalance and obesity. For more information see inflammation on page 6.	Not too high.	When it is too high! Usually as a result of poor nutrition, digestion, lack of sleep or a medical condition.	Great sleep and stress management; detoxification; hormonally balanced nutrition and supplements; exercise; additional recommendations in Chapter 11, pages 188–90 if you need extra help for managing inflammation.
Cortisol, the hormone released while under chronic stress. It has detrimental effects on our immune system, bones, brain, muscles and increases belly fat when present in excess. For more information see page 8, the section on chronic stress.	Not too high, not too low.	Excess cortisol (Chronic Stress—please understand that stress can be physical like cold temperatures, excess noise or sleep deprivation; or mental—and it doesn't matter if it is real or imagined!)	Great sleep and stress management; detoxification; hormonally balanced nutrition and supplements; exercise; additional recommendations in Chapter 11, pages 198–200 if you need help to specifically manage high cortisol.

YOUR FAT-LOSS FRIENDS

THE HORMONES THAT CONTROL YOUR APPETITE, BOOST YOUR METABOLISM AND AID FAT LOSS

FAT-LOSS FRIEND	THE PERFECT BALANCE	THE IMBALANCE THAT CAUSES FAT GAIN	THE SUPERCHARGED HORMONE DIET RECOMMENDATION THAT HELPS RESTORE BALANCE
The Hormones That Directly Stimulate Your Metabolism			
TSH, Free T3 and Free T4 are the thyroid hormones that control the metabolism of every single cell in the body. Without enough thyroid hormone, everything slows down. See more information on hypothyroidism on pages 9–10.	Not too high, not too low.	Deficiency of thyroid hormone usually as a result of nutrient deficiency, stress, toxin exposure or an immune system imbalance.	Enough sleep; stress management; sufficient calorie intake and hormonally balanced nutrition; avoidance of excessive exercise; additional recommendations in Chapter 11, pages 211–13 if you need help to specifically stimulate thyroid hormone.
Adrenaline and noradrenaline, the immediate stress-response hormones, which increase alertness and fat burning.	Not too high, not too low.	An excess of both hormones, usually as a result of stress.	Enough sleep; stress management; sufficient calorie intake and hormonally balanced nutrition; avoidance of excessive exercise; additional recommendations in Chapter 11, pages 201–2 if you need help to specifically manage stress.
Glucagon, the hormone that works opposite to insulin to boost blood sugar and encourage fat burning. It is released when our blood sugar drops (e.g., between meals) or during exercise.	Not too high, not too low.	Glucagon is too low, usually as a result of failure to eat enough protein, lack of regular exercise or excess carbohydrate consumption, which spikes insulin and blocks glucagon activity.	Hormonally balanced nutrition: specifically, avoidance of excess or unhealthy carbs, combined with the consumption of protein; and regular exercise are the best ways to stimulate glucagon release.

FAT-LOSS FRIEND	THE PERFECT BALANCE	THE IMBALANCE THAT CAUSES FAT GAIN	*THE SUPERCHARGED HORMONE DIET* RECOMMENDATION THAT HELPS RESTORE BALANCE
The Hormones That Directly Stimulate Your Metabolism (continued)			
Progesterone, the sex hormone dominant in the second half of the menstrual cycle. A deficiency of progesterone is almost always associated with PMS or fertility concerns.	Not too high, not too low.	Low progesterone in men and women, normally as a result of stress or aging.	Enough sleep; stress management; sufficient calorie intake and hormonally balanced nutrition; avoidance of excessive exercise; additional recommendations in Chapter 11, pages 207–8 if you need help to specifically increase progesterone with herbs or supplements.
The Hormones That Stimulate Fat Loss by Supporting the Growth of Metabolically Active Muscle			
DHEA, the anti-stress, anti-aging, anti-inflammatory, metabolism-enhancing hormone with masculinizing properties.	Not too high, not too low.	DHEA is too low; often as a result of stress or aging.	Enough sleep; stress management; sufficient calorie intake and hormonally balanced nutrition; avoidance of excessive exercise; additional recommendations in Chapter 11, pages 202–3 if you need help to specifically stimulate DHEA levels.
Testosterone, the masculinizing sex hormone that builds and maintains muscle. A deficiency of testosterone can prevent weight loss in both men and women even with dieting and exercise.	Not too high, not too low.	Low testosterone in men—often resulting from stress or toxin exposure. Excess testosterone in women causes weight gain, usually as a result of insulin resistance or polycystic ovary syndrome.	Great sleep and stress management; detoxification; hormonally balanced nutrition and supplements; exercise (particularly strength training); additional recommendations in Chapter 11, pages 208–10 if you need targeted help to support testosterone production.

(continued)

YOUR FAT-LOSS FRIENDS (*continued*)

THE HORMONES THAT CONTROL YOUR APPETITE, BOOST YOUR METABOLISM AND AID FAT LOSS

FAT-LOSS FRIEND	THE PERFECT BALANCE	THE IMBALANCE THAT CAUSES FAT GAIN	*THE SUPERCHARGED HORMONE DIET* RECOMMENDATION THAT HELPS RESTORE BALANCE
The Hormones That Stimulate Fat Loss by Supporting the Growth of Metabolically Active Muscle (continued)			
Growth hormone, the hormone that handles growth and repair, particularly of the bone cells, muscle cells and skin cells while we sleep. It is also released in response to exercise.	Not too high, not too low.	Growth hormone deficiency, usually as a result of poor sleep, lack of exercise, low protein intake or stress.	Enough sleep; stress management; sufficient calorie intake and hormonally balanced nutrition; regular exercise, particularly strength training; additional recommendations in Chapter 11, pages 214–16 if you need help specifically to increase growth hormone with herbs or supplements.
The Hormones That Control Your Appetite and Perform Other Functions That Fuel Fat Loss			
Melatonin, serotonin, dopamine, acetylcholine and GABA, the hormones that influence motivation, mood, sleep and cravings. See the section on depression or anxiety on page 7 to learn more about serotonin.	Not too high, not too low.	Deficiency of all of these hormones; abnormal highs and lows of dopamine are common in individuals with addictions to food, smoking, gambling, alcohol and drugs. Low serotonin is related to depression, food cravings, eating disorders, sleep disruption and anxiety.	Enough sleep; stress management; sufficient calorie intake and hormonally balanced nutrition; avoidance of excessive exercise; additional recommendations in Chapter 11, pages 193–98, 205–7, and 213–16 if you need help specifically to balance the mood hormones.

FAT-LOSS FRIEND	THE PERFECT BALANCE	THE IMBALANCE THAT CAUSES FAT GAIN	*THE SUPERCHARGED HORMONE DIET* RECOMMENDATION THAT HELPS RESTORE BALANCE
The Hormones That Control Your Appetite and Perform Other Functions That Fuel Fat Loss (continued)			
Vitamin D3 The sunshine vitamin that acts like a hormone in the body. Vitamin D supports immunity, protects us from cancer, aids weight loss and ensures success on a weight-loss program, reduces inflamma- tion, boosts mood and can help to reduce pain.	More is better.	Vitamin D3 deficiency (blood levels <125). Low vitamin D is common in individuals who live in Northern climates, cover up in the sun or use sunscreen.	Sunlight and stress management; hormonally balanced nutrition and supplements of vitamin D3. A supplement of vitamin D3 is recommended in the *Supercharged* program and beyond this 4-week plan.

What You Can Expect from *The Supercharged Hormone Diet*

In *The Hormone Diet*, I taught you that no matter how an imbalance manifests on the outside, the internal reality remains the same: *any and all* hormonal imbalance leads to difficulty losing weight, increased risk of obesity and unhealthy aging. *Balanced weight loss* is the new revolution in fat loss, and it certainly provides the answer to anyone who has ever failed at a diet and exercise program. Long-term weight loss and wellness are next to impossible until you bring your hormones back into balance.

On the 30-Day *Supercharged* program you will not only see and feel results in only 4 short weeks, you will uncover all the hormonal imbalances that are preventing you from reaching your optimal health and body composition. This means you will conclude this program with a personalized prescription for hormonal health. But we must first set your foundation for a lifetime of hormonal balance together.

Over the coming weeks you will complete a 30-day streamlined prescription for hormonal health and metabolic restoration. I have combined the perfect nutrition, supplement and exercise habits to kickstart your fat-burning hormones, quiet your fat-loss foes and balance your hormones. The primary focus of the first step of the diet plan will be detoxification, including the removal of toxic estrogen, liver detox, digestive support and reducing inflammation by removing inflammatory foods and identifying food allergies, which can absolutely block weight-loss efforts. During the first few days, you will conquer cravings, improve your digestion, gain healthy-looking skin and reduce uncomfortable belly bloat by following my detox diet. This will also begin to reset your metabolism. Your weekly exercise prescription will include two yoga sessions, four moderate cardio sessions (30 minutes maximum) and one rest day.

The second week of the detox diet is similar to the first but you have the option to add 1 serving of hypoallergenic, gluten-free grains or potatoes to your daily diet should you wish to do so. It is during the transition phase (to final stage of the diet) that you will uncover the hidden food sensitivities, which prevent you from losing weight—let alone looking and feeling your best each day. This process will allow you to begin to practice the basics of hormonally balanced nutrition, a style of eating I call the Glyci-Med approach, free of your problem foods that contribute to bloating, fatigue, water retention or pain. For instance, some Greek yogurt is a great source of protein, but not if you are allergic to dairy.

All meals in my *Supercharged* Plan are slightly higher in protein than *The Hormone Diet*. After four weeks of consuming hormone-enhancing, higher-protein meals, you are ready to ease into my approach presented in *The Carb Sensitivity Program*. Any of the 70+ recipes in this book are perfect for you at this stage of your plan. Our focus will move to metabolic support and ongoing fat loss and repair. Your weekly exercise prescription changes to include one or two yoga sessions, one or two cardio sessions (intervals) and three strength-training circuits as presented in *The Carb Sensitivity Program*.

As I previously stated in my first book, *The Hormone Diet*, if you've tried every diet and they've all failed you, *it's not your fault.* Your past efforts were doomed to fail *unless* they took into account the complex chemicals that are really running the show—your hormones!

CHAPTER 2

THE FACTORS THAT MAKE US FAT AND HORMONALLY IMBALANCED

Life is not merely to be alive, but to be well.

MARCUS VALERIUS MARTIAL

If we know that our hormones are controlling our ability to lose weight, and that all hormonal imbalances prevent us from achieving the body we desire, identifying the driving factors behind hormonal imbalance certainly makes good sense if we hope to find a lasting solution to our weight-loss challenges. In the coming weeks, we will alter your diet, exercise, sleep habits and nutrient intake to benefit your biochemistry. To do this, we first have to understand how our hormones have been negatively altered. Stress, sleep deprivation, processed foods, unhealthy digestion, tons of toxins, yo-yo dieting, pH imbalance and many other factors impact how your body processes foods, burns calories and stores fat, simply because of their hormonal effects. If you want to know why you are the way you are, keep reading.

So Much Stress

Our stress response works extremely well when there is an immediate physical stressor, such as a dangerous predator, because we can react and then quickly return to a normal balanced state once we have handled the situation. Our stress response has not yet evolved enough, however, to deal with the plentiful assortment of long-term stressors of modern-day life.

Study after study shows that stress causes abdominal fat—even in people who are otherwise thin. Researchers at Yale University, for example, found slender women who had high cortisol also had more ab fat. More results, published in the journal *Psychosomatic Medicine* in 2000, establish a link between cortisol and increased storage of, abdominal fat. I could go on to cite literally hundreds more studies that prove depression, anxiety, sleep disruption or simply feeling dissatisfied with life wreak havoc on the waistline by increasing both appetite and belly fat. The stress associated with aging and the hormonal changes of menopause also cause more ab fat. And you thought relaxing on the couch was to blame!

If all this wasn't bad enough, stress also triggers the release of appetite-stimulating hormones from the master gland in your brain, the hypothalamus.

During temporarily stressful episodes, adrenaline kicks in and taps into fat stores to provide energy to fuel the fight-or-flight response. Under prolonged periods of intense stress, however, cortisol seeks out muscle proteins for fuel instead. Over time, this attack on muscle protein leads to the destruction of metabolically active muscle tissue—tissue we need to build in order to boost metabolism and burn energy more efficiently. At the same time, the fuel released from the breakdown of muscle fiber tends to be deposited around the abdomen if it's not burned off right away. And as if our metabolism was not already in sufficient jeopardy, cortisol also comes along to inhibit the function of thyroid hormone, the master of our metabolic rate.

Over time, exposure to cortisol decreases the body's response to insulin and leads to increased insulin levels. Symptoms of this decline in insulin sensitivity include fatigue after eating carbohydrates, sugar cravings, elevated triglycerides, hypoglycemia (low blood sugar) and increased body fat at the waist, rather than at the hips or buttocks. A long-term study published in the journal *Diabetes Care* (April 2007) followed a group of women for 15 years. The women who reported feeling frequently and intensely angry, tense or stressed also showed increased risk of developing metabolic syndrome, the condition associated with insulin resistance. This study was the first to show how depressive symptoms, stressful life events, and feelings of anger or tension can be associated with high cortisol and the development of metabolic disease.

Too Short on Shut-eye

Clearly, the majority of us fail to make sleep a top priority. But women are especially guilty of putting sleep on the back burner, as evidenced by the 2007 National Sleep Foundation Poll, which focused only on the sleep habits of women. Half those polled reported that sleep and exercise are the first activities they sacrifice when they are pressed for time. The same percentage admitted they reach for foods high in sugar or carbohydrates when they feel sleepy during the day. And the cycle of weight gain continues . . .

This poll provides incredible insight into women's health, since the findings reveal women are not only sleep deprived or experiencing sleep disorders, but also carrying around excess weight. In fact, more than half the women surveyed were either overweight or obese. Women who reported experiencing sleep problems nightly were significantly more likely to be classified as obese compared with women who experienced sleep problems only a few nights a month.

A sleep schedule is vital to any weight-loss plan. Too much or too little shut-eye can add extra pounds, according to Wake Forest

University researchers who tracked study participants for 5 years. In the under-40 age group, people who slept 5 hours or less each night gained nearly two-and-a-half times as much abdominal fat as those who logged 6 to 7 hours. At the same time, those who slept 8 hours or longer added nearly twice as much belly fat as the 6- to-7-hour group. People with sleep deficits tend to eat more and use less energy because they're tired, while those who sleep too many hours a night may be less active.

Another study published in the *International Journal of Obesity* demonstrates a link between the length of time of shift work and abdominal fat. The conclusion is that chronic sleep deprivation could result in an increased risk of cardiovascular disease. The effects of sleep deprivation are similar to those seen in normal aging; therefore, sleep debt may increase the severity of age-related chronic disorders such as weight gain, elevated cholesterol or triglyceride levels and, eventually, diabetes and/or heart disease. So which comes first? Improper sleep or weight gain?

Yet another hormone impacted by sleep is melatonin. Once melatonin is released, it causes your body to cool down and sink into deeper sleep, which triggers the release of growth hormone (GH). At this point, more cell reproduction takes place and breakdown of proteins slows substantially. Essentially, your body rebuilds itself during deep sleep, especially your bone, skin and muscle cells. Since proteins are the building blocks needed for cell growth and for repair from the damaging effects of factors such as stress and ultraviolet rays, deep sleep may truly be "beauty sleep." And remember, the release of GH that occurs while we sleep is also encouraging for fat loss.

GH release naturally declines as we age, but poor quality sleep and low melatonin can cause GH production to drop off even further. Without sufficient melatonin, we lose the rejuvenating and fat-burning benefits of growth hormone and become susceptible to abdominal weight gain.

If you remember the old ad campaign of two eggs being fried with the message, "This is your brain on drugs," today we can reproduce it using sugar instead of drugs. It sounds extreme, but the average American consumes the equivalent of 152 pounds of sugar in a year. And here's the kicker, it's not only adding inches to your waistline, but setting your mood up for failure. Read on for how sugar makes you depressed.

YOUR BRAIN ON SUGAR. Once sugar (aka glucose) is ingested—whether it's in the form of a doughnut or a high-carb dinner—insulin is released. Immediately, it begins to direct the glucose in your bloodstream. Unlike fat cells, the brain can't store glucose, so this simple sugar is readily burned up upon use (a process that speeds up during times of stress, such as big meetings, or even during concentration tasks, like writing this book). Considering your brain cells need twice the energy of other cells in your body, it's no surprise then, that your head is extremely sensitive to changing blood sugar levels.

Your body also releases endorphins such as dopamine and serotonin to accompany this sugar rush, which is why, at first, you'll feel happier, and perhaps even calmer. However, these receptor sites slow production to regulate the same endorphins that had you feeling so good, causing a crash in mood and even depression—and so the cycle begins and we reach for more sugar.

In fact, patients who were treated for both type 2 diabetes and depression at the same time achieve better results, according to a new study by researchers from the University of Pennsylvania. This is one of the many reasons I include dietary changes for every patient that comes into my office with concerns of depression and/or mood swings.

THE SWEET TOOTH—UNVEILED. What goes up (in this case, blood sugar) must come down. Sleepiness right after a sugar-rich meal is a classic symptom of reduced insulin sensitivity (which down the road leads to diabetes), along with a dip in mood and energy. I find most patients in my practice with high insulin have low levels of serotonin—the "happy" hormone that controls our mood, sleep patterns, self-esteem, ability to make decisions and cravings. According to research from Princeton University, "food addiction" evolves as a result of changes in brain pathways. Sugar causes the release of the hormone dopamine in the brain— the same response activated by addictive drugs. These chemical adaptations cause changes in dopamine release over time. In this particular study, rats actually became sugar-dependent, paving the way for theories that sugar can be physiologically addictive. The rats even experienced 'withdrawals' through low levels of dopamine and anxiety. They displayed chattering teeth and were reluctant to leave their homes—except if it was to get more sugar. Given this, it's not hard to believe that in brain scans, sugar appears to be as addictive as cocaine.

THE PROOF IS IN THE (SUGAR-FILLED) PUDDING. Research suggests that drinking sweetened beverages, even diet drinks, is associated with an increased risk of depression. People who drank more than 4 cans or cups per day of soda were 30 percent more likely to develop depression than those who drank no soda. Those who drank 4 cans of fruit punch per day were about 38 percent more likely to develop depression than those who did not drink sweetened drinks. Not to mention that these drinks often lack any essential nutrients and healthy brain fuel. A similar study in the *British Journal of Psychiatry* (of more than 3,400 middle-aged civil servants) found that those who had a diet containing a lot of processed foods—ranging from desserts to refined grains— had a 58 percent increased risk for depression, whereas those whose diet could be described as containing more whole foods— think vegetables, fruits and fish—had a reduced risk for depression of 26 percent.

In a nutshell, the right amount of quality sleep actually helps you to lose weight by influencing the hormones that control your appetite, increase your metabolism and reduce your stress levels. The better you sleep, the less your stress; the less your stress, the better your brain power, appetite control and, ultimately, your body composition.

Poor Nutrition Habits

Just think how our eating habits have evolved with our busy lifestyle. We shovel in a fast bite at our desk, in the car or standing over the kitchen counter so we can quickly move on with work or run errands. We eat late at night in front of the TV, or we skip meals altogether. Think about our food choices. Packaged, processed convenience foods loaded with hidden salt, fat and sugar. Yeesh! These foods not only do a number on our waistlines, but also wreak havoc on our digestion. Here's my summary of the nutrition no-nos, their hormonal effects and their long-term outcomes.

NASTY NUTRITION HABIT THAT CAUSES HORMONAL IMBALANCES	METABOLIC EFFECTS OF THE HORMONAL IMBALANCE	IMMEDIATE CONSEQUENCES AND LONG-TERM RISKS
What We Eat		
Inflammatory foods such as trans fats, processed sugar and white flours; excess red meats and full-fat dairy products; processed meats and vegetable oils (cottonseed, soy and excess safflower or sunflower oil)	• Increased blood sugar, insulin and inflammatory markers • Poor appetite control and increased cravings	Insulin resistance, heart disease, diabetes, cancer, obesity, Alzheimer's disease
Meats and dairy products laden with growth hormone, steroid hormones and antibiotic residues	• Elevated growth hormone • Harmful excess of estrogen, progesterone and testosterone	Increased risk of obesity; greater risk of breast, prostate and uterine cancers; estrogen dominance

NASTY NUTRITION HABIT	METABOLIC EFFECTS	IMMEDIATE & LONG-TERM EFFECTS
High-fructose corn syrup products	• Increased appetite and cravings • Increased blood sugar and insulin	Spikes in appetite, overeating, insulin resistance, obesity
Fat-free products	• Increased appetite and cravings • Increased blood sugar and insulin	Spikes in appetite, overeating, insulin resistance and weight gain
Artificial sweeteners and sugar-free products	• Increased appetite and cravings • Increased blood sugar and insulin • Increased weight gain	Spikes in appetite, overeating, insulin resistance and weight gain
Excess alcohol	• Increased insulin • Decreased testosterone • Increased harmful estrogen	Insulin resistance, estrogen dominance, symptoms of low testosterone such as loss of muscle and increased fat gain
Low fiber intake	• Increased blood sugar and insulin • Poor appetite control • Increased cravings • Weight gain • Increased harmful estrogen	Insulin resistance, diabetes, heart disease, colon cancer, breast cancer, prostate cancer, obesity
When and How We Eat		
Overeating (super-sizing)	• Increased blood sugar and insulin • Increased cortisol (stress hormone)	Excess appetite, more overeating, insulin resistance and weight gain
Skipping breakfast	• Increased cortisol • Decreased thyroid hormone and, therefore, lower metabolic rate • Increased cravings • Tendency to overeat later in the day • Increased appetite	Spikes in appetite, overeating, slower metabolism and weight gain

NASTY NUTRITION HABIT	METABOLIC EFFECTS	IMMEDIATE & LONG-TERM EFFECTS
Late-night eating	• Increased blood sugar and insulin • Decreased melatonin • Decreased growth hormone	Poor sleep quality, excess appetite, overeating, excess cortisol the following day, weight gain
Insufficient calories	• Increased cortisol • Decreased thyroid hormone and, therefore, lower metabolic rate	Excess appetite, overeating, slower metabolism and weight gain
Stress-related eating	• Increased insulin • Increased cortisol • Increased appetite and cravings	Excess appetite, overeating, insulin resistance and weight gain
Failing to balance protein, carbohydrates and fats	• Increased blood sugar and insulin • Increased cortisol • Poor appetite control • Increased cravings • Increased estrogen in men; increased testosterone in women	Insulin resistance, estrogen dominance, abdominal weight gain, heart disease, diabetes, increased risk of cancer
Cooking on high heats	• Increased cell damage and inflammation	Insulin resistance, heart disease, diabetes, cancer, obesity, Alzheimer's disease

Bad Belly Blues

Unhealthy digestion contributes to obesity and is a potential source of troublesome inflammation and hormone disruption. I'll bet you didn't know that your digestive system is one of the largest sites of hormone production in the body and that your hormones influence your digestion, just as your digestion influences your hormones. Next to correcting sleep problems, digestive health and liver detoxification are the most commonly overlooked aspects of a successful fat-loss program, and this is precisely why step 1 of the detox diet contains only anti-inflammatory and hypoallergenic foods.

According to statistics from the National Digestive Diseases Information Clearinghouse (NDDIC), over 60 million Americans are affected by digestive disease. No wonder curing tummy troubles has exploded into $107-billion-a-year industry in the United States! Even though I see digestive issues every day in my clinical practice, I am nonetheless astounded by these statistics. An awful lot of people have very unhappy bellies.

Consider just a few of the afflictions:

- **Gastroesophageal Reflux Disease (GERD)**—Also known as acid reflux, this uncomfortable condition affects 20 percent of the US population and 29 percent of the Canadian population.
- **Lactose Intolerance**—An inability to digest the sugars in dairy products affects approximately 75 percent of the adult population worldwide.
- **Constipation**—More than a million prescriptions are doled out each year just to help people "get moving."
- **Gallstones**—More than half a million gallbladder removal surgeries are performed each year to cure this painful problem.
- **Gastritis**—Almost 4 million people suffer from conditions associated with gastric inflammation; over 2 million prescriptions are written annually for gastritis.
- **Dyspepsia/Upset Stomach**—Each year more than 8 million people endure chronic or recurrent pain in the upper abdomen.
- **Hemorrhoids**—More than 8 million people experience this painful inflammation.
- **Diarrhea**—Eight to 12 million people visit the doctor annually for this problem.
- **Irritable Bowel Syndrome (IBS)**—More than 2 million people are pained by IBS; 46,000 are on disability because of it.
- **Peptic Ulcers**—Two million prescriptions are written for ulcers yearly.

Should these numbers really surprise us? We are overstressed, overtired and undernourished. No wonder our digestive systems are mounting a major protest. This intricate system is critical for hormonal balance because it controls its own functions via hormonal signals. Amazingly, over 30 hormone genes are currently known to be expressed in the stomach and the intestines, making your *gut* the largest endocrine organ in your body! While we usually think of the digestive system as an entity that resides in our bellies, it actually involves both the nervous system *and* the cells and activities of the endocrine system. Your nervous system, especially the parasympathetic (rest-and-digest) and sympathetic (fight-or-flight), has exerts a powerful influence on your digestion. However, your digestive system has its own nervous system too. In fact, it has just as many nerves as your spinal cord! So when you get a gut instinct, *go with it.*

One aspect of digestive health that has a direct impact on your potential for hormonal balance is your gut flora, which plays a key role in the breakdown of excess estrogen. The trouble is, we are constantly bombarded these days by commercial messages urging us to fight germs and rid ourselves of bacteria. But in the right places and amounts, bacteria are essential to our health and wellness. These beneficial bacteria, also called probiotics, exist in the digestive tract.

Under normal circumstances, friendly bacteria found in our digestive system live with us in symbiotic harmony. But factors such as poor diet, and medications such as birth control pills, antibiotics and corticosteroids, can upset this healthy balance and lead to a host of difficulties, including increased body fat storage and estrogen dominance. Research completed at the Department of Genomic Sciences at the University of Washington found increased fat storage in rats that lacked probiotics. The correct balance of intestinal flora seems to limit fat storage by repressing the expression of a protein called fasting-induced adipocyte factor (FIAF).

At least you can take comfort in knowing that the simple suggestions in *The Supercharged Hormone Diet* can help you solve just about any digestive debacle for good. Plus, you can lose weight while doing it!

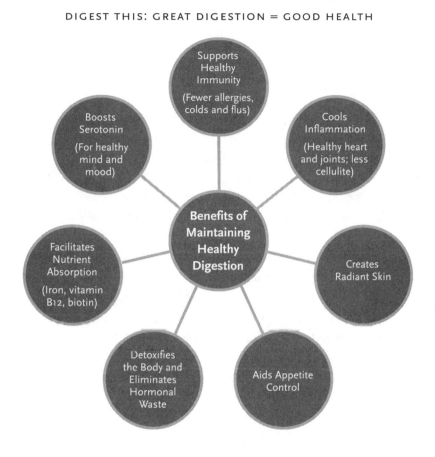

Body Toxicity and Environmental Toxins

Without even realizing it, we are constantly exposed to toxins that have the potential to disrupt our hormones and cause weight gain. Several toxins in our environment cause estrogenic activity and lower testosterone, which result in obesity and fertility concerns. The phthalates, dioxins and bisphenols found in plastics are especially troublesome.

Your thyroid is also particularly sensitive to chlorine, fluoride, mercury, pesticides and other toxins. These types of chemicals have been shown to disrupt communication between the hypothalamus, pituitary and thyroid—the pathway that closely controls our metabolic rate. When researchers looked at the effects of synthetic chemicals such as DDT, phenol derivatives, phthalates, polyhalogenated hydrocarbons, amitrole and thiocarbamates on the thyroid, they noticed thyroid suppression.

It's clear: toxins inhibit your thyroid, the master of your metabolic rate, which in turn leads to weight gain. According to Dr. Mark Schauss, toxins can *lower* an individual's body temperature and resting metabolic rate by as much as 7 percent. A direct link between chemicals called phthalates and thyroid hormone levels was confirmed by the University of Michigan. Higher concentrations of urinary phthalate metabolites and BPA were associated with greater impacts on serum thyroid measures. Here's the kicker: As urinary metabolite concentrations increased, serum levels of certain thyroid hormone levels decreased. So if you are feeling fat, frumpy and forgetful from a sluggish thyroid, the culprit may be lurking closely in your headquarters, particularly your kitchen.

Your thyroid isn't the only hormone that takes a hit from too many toxins. Researchers at the University of Rochester Medical Center have now linked the drop in testosterone caused by phthalates to abdominal obesity, insulin resistance and the onset of type 2 diabetes in men. Meanwhile the state of sperm in our society is dropping. According to *Internet Journal of Urology*, the average sperm count fell from 113 million per milliliter in 1940 to 66 million in 1990. In addition, the definition of a "normal" sperm count fell from 60 million per milliliter to 20 million in the same period. Phthalates, in particular, have been connected to reproductive problems in baby boys, smaller penis sizes, testicular problems in adolescents and reduced testosterone production in men.

While testosterone is dropping in men, our estrogen is increasing in women (and men!). It's a given that not all estrogen is bad, however, you certainly don't want to put out the welcome mat for this guest as it can contribute to PMS, lower body fat, cellulite, endometriosis, uterine cysts, certain cancers and even reduced thyroid function. In our male counterparts, it can contribute to breast enlargement, lower sperm counts, reduced libido and the list goes on. We are constantly exposed to estrogen-like compounds in foods that contain toxic pesticides, herbicides and growth hormones.

So where are all these toxins setting up shop? Unfortunately your fat cells are the perfect host. Your main weapon against this toxic surge—your liver—must continually metabolize, detoxify and excrete hormone breakdown products via the bile into the digestive tract for removal from the body. So it's essential to keep it working optimally.

Yo-yo Dieting and Long-Term Excessive Calorie Restriction

When your caloric intake bounces up and down, your metabolism suffers through a dangerous series of highs and lows. The end result of this havoc includes weight gain (exactly what you did *not* want), mood changes, cravings, the loss of precious metabolically active muscle tissue and, ultimately, a damaged metabolism.

The short-term victories achieved with this type of eating are *always* followed with rebound weight gain because of the loss of muscle and, whether we like it or not, our hormones will kick in to return the body to status quo. Furthermore, the spike in stress hormones caused by excessive caloric restriction is highly destructive and will actually cause you to want to eat and eat . . . and eat some more. This type of caloric restriction can ravage both your hormonal balance and your metabolism. But here's the really scary bit: repeatedly losing and gaining weight is also linked to cardiovascular disease, stroke, diabetes and altered immune function. A weight-loss program that compromises muscle while you lose fat is metabolically harmful and serves only to speed the aging process. Not what you are looking for, I'm sure.

So exactly how much damage can that oh-so-low-calorie diet do? An older study in the *Journal of Clinical Endocrinology & Metabolism* (1976) discovered that total fasting reduction in a 53 percent reduction in serum T3 levels (your active thyroid hormone) and a reciprocal 58 percent increase in reverse T3 levels (which blocks thyroid hormone). In a given day, your liver converts the less active form of your thyroid hormone, T4, to reverse T3 as a way of getting rid of excess T3. But in a low calorie situation where your body needs to conserve energy, the percentage may spike significantly, and as you can see from the numbers above it's not unusual to find yourself converting 50 percent or more of your essential thyroid hormone into inert metabolic wastage. Opposite to the drop in thyroid, we also experience a significant increase in cortisol during a starvation diet—it is the acute stress alone that activates this surge (remember, as far as your body is concerned it is under the impression that there is now less food available). Together, this hormonal shift doesn't exactly render itself well on the scale and you can imagine how it can set you up for a rebound as your body struggles to restore its former state of homeostasis.

Safe fat loss means losing only fat, while preserving muscle. A healthy, long-term solution means avoiding severe caloric restrictions or fad diet approaches that are unsustainable and always result in hormonally driven rebound weight gain, not to mention the discouragement that comes with feeling like you've failed.

Remember, your body and your hormones are programmed to work against extreme diets by increasing your appetite and slowing your metabolic rate when you cut too many calories. When your metabolism drops, you gain weight and feel tired and sluggish. On the other hand, when you use the right weight-loss techniques, your metabolism gets an energizing boost that leaves you feeling brighter and looking your best. These facts are exactly why I have elaborated on the importance of a cheat meal for maintaining your metabolism in Chapter 10.

pH Imbalance

Although the stomach should contain plenty of acid to do its job effectively, a slightly alkaline environment is optimal everywhere else to allow the body's metabolic, enzymatic, immunologic and repair mechanisms to function at their best. pH imbalance interferes with the activity of our hormones and our ability to lose weight. The most common pH abnormality is an acidic body pH (pH < 7.0). To maximize the results of your 4-week program, your pH must be restored.

The most common form of pH imbalance outside the stomach is *excess acidity*. This condition has become prevalent today because a poor diet, insufficient exercise and chronic stress can lead to excess acid in our internal environment. Specifically, high-protein foods, processed cereals and flours, sugar, coffee, tea and alcohol are acidifying, while vegetables, millet, soy, almonds and wild rice are alkalinizing.

You will enjoy the most dramatic results from this program when your body is slightly alkaline. Acidity decreases your body's ability to absorb the vitamins and minerals from your foods and supplements, interferes with your ability to detoxify, disrupts your metabolism and makes you more prone to fatigue and mood changes. For all these reasons, I have included pH testing as part of the Best Body Assessment outlined in the next chapter.

Harmful Hormones in Our Foods

Hormones are often used in farming to make animals grow more quickly or to increase milk production in cattle. There are six steroid hormones currently approved by the US Food and Drug Administration (FDA) for use in food production: estradiol, progesterone, testosterone, zeranol, trenbolone acetate and melengestrol acetate. Zeranol, trenbolone acetate and melengestrol acetate are anabolic steroids used to make animals grow faster and larger. Current federal regulations allow the use of these hormones for growing cattle and sheep but not poultry (chickens, turkeys and ducks) or pigs. Much of the controversy surrounds beef, since hormones are given to more than 90 percent of beef cattle in the United States.

The FDA also allows the use of the protein hormone rbGH (bovine growth hormone) to increase milk production in dairy cattle. This substance is not approved for use in dairy cattle in Canada and Europe, however, because of concerns for both animal welfare and human health. The use of rbGH increases insulin-like growth factor-1 (IGF-1) in the milk of treated cows as much as tenfold. Though IGF-1 naturally occurs in humans and cows, higher than normal levels of this substance have recently been linked to breast and prostate cancers in humans. To date, no studies show drinking milk with high IGF-1 causes levels of this hormone to increase in humans, but researchers do know IGF-1 can be absorbed into the bloodstream from our digestive tract. Who wants to take the chance?

To make matters worse, increased milking can make hormone-treated cows more prone to mastitis, a bacterial inflammation of the udder. Residues from the antibiotics used to treat the cows then end up in the milk we drink. In the previous section you learned about the importance of healthy bacterial balance in the gut. Antibiotic residues from cow's milk can definitely disrupt the delicate and very necessary balance in our digestive tract.

Steroid hormones are also problematic additions to our foods. Both estradiol and progesterone are considered probable carcinogens when added to foods by the National Toxicology Program at the US National Institutes of Health. Even though the US FDA has concluded that the amount of hormone residue in our food is negligible compared with the amount the body produces naturally, many health experts agree that any excess is too much. Estrogen has been linked with breast cancer in women; testosterone with prostate cancer in men. Progesterone has been found to increase the growth of ovarian, breast and uterine tumors. Rather than taking chances with our health, we can certainly opt for hormone-free organic meat and dairy products instead.

In 1989, the European Union issued a ban on all meat from animals treated with steroid and growth hormones—a ban that is still in effect today. While Canada does not allow any growth hormone use in animals, steroid hormones are still permitted for beef cattle.

Toxins in Our Medicine Cabinet

While they are designed to help our health, many medications are a source of toxins and hormonal disruption. The biggest culprits are antidepressants, birth control pills, synthetic HRT and corticosteroids. Yes, these medications have a role to play in certain instances, but I encourage you to consider trying a natural alternative first. Specifically, I strongly recommend that you fully understand the side effects and long-term risks of any and all medications you choose to use.

When these types of drugs are in your system, total hormonal balance becomes much more difficult to achieve. The birth control pill, in particular, contains much higher levels of hormones than even conventional hormone replacement therapy (HRT), which has already been proven to increase a woman's breast cancer risk. Antidepressant medications interfere with the liver's detoxification pathways, described later on in Chapter 4, the detox chapter. These pathways are involved with the breakdown and elimination of harmful toxins, and when they are not functioning at their best, more toxins accumulate, which then upsets our metabolism. I explain to patients that this process is like mixing alcohol with antidepressant medications. The effects of alcohol are more pronounced while taking one of these medications because of the interference with the detox pathways in the liver. The liver simply does not metabolize and break down the alcohol as quickly. As a result, you will feel the effects of alcohol faster and more intensely while taking an antidepressant medication. Please note that I provide this only as an example of the metabolic effects of antidepressants and not as a means of encouraging you to stop taking any depression meds.

Don't Worry, Be Healthy

A lack of exercise and poor diet are obvious causes of weight gain, but I'll bet you never thought about all these other factors that could be blocking your success at fat loss. We just looked at quite a list of offenders! Over time, these factors cause conditions of long-term imbalance—and may result in one of the eight most common fat-packing hormonal imbalances we discussed in the last chapter. In fact, I suspect it is one of these conditions that has enticed you to pick up this book in the first place. But I hope you now realize that if you haven't been successful at achieving or maintaining your fat-loss goals before, *the problem may not be your fault.*

Here's my promise to you: all of these factors can be improved upon. Better health and hormonal balance can be experienced within just days of making a few simple changes! Let's get you started.

"Doing the Hormone Diet this year was one of the smartest and best things my husband and I have ever done. We both feel so much better now that we have lost weight and, more importantly, learned how to shop and eat properly. What we thought were healthy eating choices were actually not. The program taught us to read labels and introduced us to many delicious and healthy foods, some of which we had never even heard of! We also followed the workouts, and we were pleasantly surprised to see such great results after having only half-hour sessions as opposed to working out in a gym for hours. For approximately 10 years, I used my treadmill faithfully and never lost one pound. If only I had known then what I know today!

"Not only have we lost weight and inches, but I have also stopped using one of my blood pressure medications and hopefully will be off my cholesterol meds in the near future. My hair loss even stopped and many of my previous complaints disappeared. Overall, the program was easy to follow and the benefits have been amazing. We would strongly recommend this program to anyone, and we are looking forward to showing off our new bodies this summer!"

NIRVANA

STATS	JAN	MAR	LOST
Weight	162.8	154.4	8.4
Fat Mass	63.5	49.9	13.6
Body Fat	39%	32%	7%
BP	134/91	119/82	↓
Waist (inches)	35.5	34.5	1
Hips (inches)	44	40	4

(continued)

INITIAL CHIEF COMPLAINTS:

1. Overweight
2. Health issues (too many medications)
3. Anxiety, stress
4. High blood pressure and high cholesterol
5. Hair loss

DENNIS

STATS	JAN	MAR	LOST
Weight	239.4	219.2	20.2
Lean Body Mass	160.9	163.3	+ 2.4
Fat Mass	78.5	55.9	22.6
Body Fat	32%	26%	6%
BP	137/95	132/77	↓
Waist (inches)	43	40.25	2.75

INITIAL CHIEF COMPLAINTS:

1. Overweight
2. Lack of energy
3. Work-related stress
4. Poor sleep habits
5. Lack of focus

CHAPTER 3

THE BEST BODY ASSESSMENT:
SETTING YOUR HORMONAL HEALTH
AND WELLNESS GOALS

Nothing great was ever achieved without enthusiasm.

RALPH WALDO EMERSON

To effectively measure your progress over the coming weeks, you need to begin by assessing where you are today. Establishing your body composition and full range of body benchmarks now will help you monitor your progress over the next 30 days far more than simply watching the number on your scale. Before you embark on your *supercharged* program, I encourage you to measure several variables, which can be easily done right at home with these tools:

1. A camera to take before and after pictures of yourself. You can send us your before and after pictures along with your full stats through drnatashaturner.com once you have completed the *Supercharged* Hormone Diet.
2. Litmus paper pH-testing strips from your local health-food store (or available through my website, as part of the Hormone Diet Basic Detox Kit).
3. A tape measure.
4. A digital scale.
5. A watch that measures seconds or a heart rate monitor.
6. A means of measuring your body fat is optional, but you can purchase a scale with this option already built in. Visit tanita.com for information on obtaining a home-use scale that

measures body-fat percentage. If you cannot afford one, don't worry. The rest of the Best Body Assessment measurements will still provide a very good indication of your overall health.

7. If you have high blood pressure, I strongly suggest investing in a BP monitor to use at home daily.

When you have all the tools you need, you're ready to complete your Best Body Assessment:

1. **Take your before picture at the beginning and your after picture at the end of the program.** Keep these handy because we want you to share them with us on drnatashaturner.com. Your success stories will help to inspire others, just like those I have included in this book to inspire you.

2. **Determine your body composition.** Safe weight loss means preserving precious muscle tissue and losing fat. During weight loss, far too many of us fixate on the numbers on our scale. We can avoid this unhealthy trap by understanding that a handful of muscle actually weighs more than the same-size handful of fat. Remember this concept when you feel frustrated because the number on your scale just won't seem to budge. Instead, judge your progress by all of the body composition values listed here, by how your clothes fit and—most importantly—how you look and feel.

   • Weigh yourself while naked, first thing in the morning on an empty stomach after going to the bathroom, and record your body weight.
     Start date: _____
     End of 30 days: _____
   • Waist measurement (remember, measurements should be less than 40 inches for men; less than 35 inches for women). The measurements should be taken at your belly button. Or more specifically, your waist size should

be less than half your height (measured in inches).
Start date: _____
End of 30 days: _____

- Hip measurement (around the widest part of your hips).
Start date: _____
End of 30 days: _____

- Calculate your waist-hip ratio by dividing your waist measurement by your hip measurement (ideal waist-hip ratio is < 0.9 for men; < 0.8 for women). See page 44 for instructions.
Start date: _____
End of 30 days: _____

- If possible, measure your body-fat percentage via a scale, either at home or at a local health club, first thing in the morning on an empty stomach.
Start date: _____
End of 30 days: _____

- If possible (meaning if your body-fat measuring machine is able to provide this information), record your lean body mass, which pertains to your muscle and bone mass. You will want to see this value remain the same or increase.
Start date: _____
End of 30 days: _____

In addition to measuring your body-fat percentage, you should also consider *where* your stubborn fat pockets are located, since your hormones dictate where fat is stored in your body. Assess your shape and note the areas that are currently of concern. You will want to pay attention to these spots as well as the areas noted on page 43 as you progress through the 30-day *Supercharged* plan and the months after the program.

(continued on page 45)

Measuring your muscle mass is important because good muscle tone has many additional benefits, even when the body is completely at rest. These include

- **A major metabolic boost.** With the help of your thyroid hormones, muscle tissue dictates your metabolic rate.

  Fat is far less metabolically active than muscle, which means the more fat you have, the fewer calories you need to maintain your weight. As a result, it is much easier to gain unwanted weight when you have insufficient muscle simply because you are less likely to use all the calories you take in each day and more likely to store the excess calories as fat. This is also why some men, who naturally have a higher ratio of muscle to fat, tend to burn up what they eat faster, although an overweight man may have a slower metabolism compared with a slim woman with more muscle tissue.

- **Increase in insulin sensitivity.** Muscle cells are important targets for the action of insulin, since most of our insulin receptors are present within muscle tissue. As we age and naturally lose muscle, the risk of insulin resistance increases. When our cells lose their sensitivity to insulin, more of this hormone must be produced in order for it to do its job, which means more of the hormonal signal to store fat is present in our system.

One pound of muscle and 1 pound of fat are NOT the same size.

One pound of muscle on a scale and 1 pound of fat on a scale *both* weigh 1 pound. The difference is in *total volume and density.* One pound of muscle is compact and is typically about the size of a baseball. One pound of fat, however, is about three times the size and has an amorphous, jelly-like appearance.

FAT-STORAGE SITE	PROBLEM AREA FOR YOU?	POSSIBLE HORMONAL INTERPRETATION	
		HORMONAL IMBALANCE— MEN	HORMONAL IMBALANCE— WOMEN
Belly or abdomen (apple shape)		High estrogen Low testosterone High cortisol High insulin Low growth hormone	Low estrogen (menopause) High estrogen (premenopausal) High testosterone High cortisol High insulin Low growth hormone
Back of the arm (triceps)		High insulin Low DHEA	High insulin Low DHEA
Hips/buttocks/ hamstrings (pear shape)		High estrogen	High estrogen Low progesterone
Love handles (above the hips)		Insulin and blood sugar imbalance	Insulin and blood sugar imbalance
Chest (over the pectoral muscles)		High estrogen (Often coupled with high insulin and low testosterone)	High estrogen
Back ("bra fat")		High insulin	High testosterone High insulin
Thighs		Low growth hormone	Low growth hormone High estrogen

Abdominal fat fuels hormonal imbalance just as hormonal imbalance fuels abdominal fat. It's tough to say which sets in first, but research firmly establishes that those of us who tend to accumulate pounds around the waist (apple shape) have a higher risk of heart disease, diabetes and high blood pressure than those who carry excess weight on the hips and thighs (pear shape).

One of the quickest ways to determine whether you are hormonally imbalanced is to measure your waist-hip ratio (WHR). Calculating your WHR determines definitively whether the weight around your midsection exceeds that surrounding your hips and thighs.

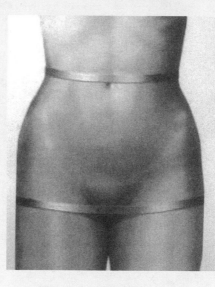

WAIST-HIP MEASUREMENT

Measure your waist at your belly button. Measure your hips around the widest part of your buttocks. A waist measurement of more than 35 inches for women or more than 40 inches for men is pushing into the unhealthy range. Next, calculate your WHR by dividing the measurement of your waist by the measurement of your hips. If your WHR is greater than 0.9 for men or 0.8 for women, you are also at risk.

Example: Let's say Mary's waist measures 28 inches and her hips are 33 inches. Her waist-to-hip ratio would be calculated as follows: 28 ÷ 33 = 0.84 (71 ÷ 84 = 0.84). Because 0.8 is considered unsafe for women, Mary is at risk and needs to lose some belly fat.

3. **Check your body pH.** Acidity in the whole body (outside the stomach) is a major cause of hormonal imbalance. Hormones function best at a neutral to slightly alkaline pH. Test your body fluids (saliva or urine) using litmus paper strips purchased from your local health-food store, or as part of the Hormone Diet Basic Detox Kit, first thing in the morning or 1 hour before a meal or 2 hours after eating. Before brushing your teeth, fill your

mouth with saliva and swallow; repeat; then spit directly on the pH test strip. This three-step process will ensure a clean saliva sample. Measure your saliva pH in the same manner again later in the day, at least 2 hours after eating. Match your strip to the associated color on the package of pH papers to determine your body pH. Ideally, your pH strip matched with 7.2 to 7.4 on the package (usually dark green or bluish, depending on the brand of pH papers).

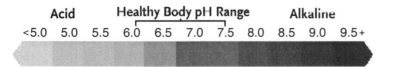

Acid	Healthy Body pH Range		Alkaline		
<5.0 5.0 5.5	6.0 6.5 7.0 7.5	8.0	8.5 9.0 9.5+		

If your values are abnormal, continue to measure and record your pH daily on your wellness tracker. Otherwise, testing once a week will suffice.

4. **Measure your blood pressure (BP) and your heart rate.**

BP: If you do not have a monitor at home, check your BP at your local pharmacy or your doctor's office. Optimal BP is 110/70, with the high range being 120/80. This number should not increase with age. Monitor your blood pressure daily, if you currently have high blood pressure or are at risk. If you find your BP is mildly elevated, add a supplement of potassium (99 mg/day) and additional magnesium (200 to 500 mg at bedtime based on bowel tolerance) to your supplement regimen.

Start date: _____

End of 30 days: _____

Resting heart rate: You may do this by recording your pulse as soon as you awaken, *before you get out of bed*. Measure your pulse for 15 seconds, then multiply the number by 4 to calculate your heartbeats per minute. Note that if your pulse increases from one week to the next, you may be overexercising.

Start date: _____

End of 30 days: _____

The Three Keys to Success

For any lifestyle change or weight-loss program to be successful, three key elements need to be present: **commitment, planning/ organization** and **motivation**. You have just set some of your body composition and wellness goals through the Best Body Assessment, but here's a nice summary checklist.

The Hormone Diet Goal-setting Checklist

Please check off any of the goals below that you would like to achieve:

Lose body fat ☐

Increase lean muscle ☐

Improve body composition ☐

Improve nutrition/diet ☐

Enhance vitality ☐

Improve sex drive ☐

Improve digestion ☐

Eliminate gas/bloating ☐

Detoxify or improve liver health ☐

Eliminate hypoglycemia ☐

Eliminate cravings ☐

Control appetite ☐

Improve energy ☐

Improve sleep ☐

Balance mood ☐

Reduce pain/inflammation ☐

Improve immune system ☐

Commit to regular exercise ☐

Improve cardiovascular fitness ☐

Increase strength ☐

Improve skin ☐

Reduce fine lines/wrinkles ☐

Achieve healthier/shinier hair ☐

Balance hormones ☐

Enhance memory ☐

Improve concentration ☐

Reduce risk of cancer ☐

Reduce risk of osteoporosis ☐

Reduce risk of heart disease/stroke ☐

Prevent Alzheimer's disease ☐

Other goals: _____

_____

_____

_____

In the rest of this book, I have provided you with all of the planning and organizational tools you will need. Now all you have to do is commit to your goals.

Commitment Agreement to Your New Hormonally Balanced Lifestyle

You are about to make a commitment to a healthier, hormonally balanced lifestyle that will enable you to lose fat, gain strength and live younger longer. The journey will take a lot of discipline, determination and hard work. You're feeling energized and ready to start. That's great because your enthusiasm will help you stay motivated. But, over the next few weeks, there will be times when you may feel frustrated, fatigued, stressed or confused. You may want to make excuses or even give up. It will be during those times that you will have to focus on your initial goals and on why you decided to do this program in the first place. Go back and review your goals regularly to help you stay on track. Remember, the pain and frustration of the process will be entirely worth it when the end result is a completely new, transformed, healthier *you*!

This book will coach you through the program, but no one can get you any healthier than you want to be and only you can follow through on the commitment. So are you ready to start?

I, _____

- Promise that before I give up on my goals, I'll sit down and re-read this commitment.
- Promise I will keep a record of everything I eat using the wellness tracker in this book.
- Promise to remember what I am trying to achieve when I'm tempted to cheat.
- Promise to commit to the program and will not quit until I reach my body composition and hormonal health goals.

- Promise to reward myself regularly with a non-food-related treat such as:_____

  _____

  _____

  _____

Signed:_____

Date:_____

Congratulations, you have made the commitment!
The results you will see and feel will serve as your ongoing source of motivation. Good luck!

"It was my last attempt to gain control over my body! The Hormone Diet is and continues to be very successful for me. At the age of 54, I have tried it all. I needed to gain control over my hormonal imbalance and my weight. Dr. Turner's approach is a holistic one. I learned to read my body and to gain insight into the foods I eat. She taught me how to be a better consumer of health care and how to shop better for healthy foods."

SUSAN

STATS	JAN	MAY	LOST
Weight	143.2	141	2.2
Lean Body Mass	95.5	111.4	+15.9
Fat Mass	47.7	29.6	18.1
Body Fat	33%	21%	12%
BP	118/81	116/78	↓
Waist (inches)	36	33	3
Hips (inches)	41.5	39.75	1.75

INITIAL CHIEF COMPLAINTS:

1. Hot flashes
2. Hair thinning
3. Poor sleep
4. Asthma

CHAPTER 4

THE *SUPERCHARGED* HORMONE DIET: DETOX—STEP 1 AND TRANSITION PHASES

He who has health, has hope. And he who has hope, has everything.

ARABIAN PROVERB

Good health, weight-loss success and hormonal balance are intimately connected to optimal liver function. But over time our organ functions can become sluggish. In really basic terms, think of your liver as a motor that runs best when regularly provided with only the very best fuel. We simply must complete a liver and bowel detox to restore hormonal balance and prepare your body for safe weight loss.

Your liver can also provide quick energy when necessary by releasing sugar stores (glycogen), *if* it's functioning optimally. Low blood sugar (hypoglycemia) is common in people with liver disease because this vital organ is unable to perform its task successfully. If you have an underfunctioning liver or liver disease, you may also have three times as much sugar in your blood after consuming carbs than someone with a normally functioning liver. This blood sugar imbalance can lead to insulin resistance, low energy, fatty liver, obesity and other long-term health risks. Since tissues in the brain and central nervous system rely solely on sugar for energy, they too become highly vulnerable when the liver is damaged or underperforming.

The Detox Pathways in Your Liver

Regardless of their source, all toxins must be processed through the body via the detoxification pathways in the liver. Liver detoxification consists of two phases designed to allow potentially toxic compounds to be converted into water-soluble forms that can be easily excreted into the bile for passage through the digestive tract as waste or filtered through the kidneys.

Phase I is the phase that turns toxic compounds into water-soluble products. During this process, enzymes add an oxygen molecule to the toxin to make free radicals, which are often more toxic than the original substance. Throughout Phase I, the nutrients copper, magnesium, zinc and vitamin C are essential to protect liver cells and prevent free radicals from causing damage.

Phase II focuses on neutralizing the products from Phase I by adding another substance that makes elimination through the kidneys or bile easier. After passing through Phase II, the original substance becomes completely water soluble, allowing it to be excreted from the body. Phase II uses its own set of enzymes, many of which require sulfur-containing amino acids (methionine, taurine and cysteine), other nutrients (glycine, glutamine, choline and inositol) and antioxidants (glutathione, vitamin E, coenzyme Q10, vitamin C and lipoic acid). This step is vitally important to the breakdown and elimination of hormonal waste products.

These two phases are intimately related and should ideally take place at the same rate. The great news is the *Supercharged* Hormone Diet detox plan supports the process beautifully. Along with the detoxifying foods you will enjoy, the detox supplements and shakes recommended daily also provide all of the vitamins, minerals and amino acids necessary to support your liver detoxification pathways. And the very best part: get ready to experience no cravings! This is the most common feedback that I receive in my practice—cravings clear up, troublesome preoccupations with food end and energy levels increase!

Healthy Digestion Does Your Body Good

Next to correcting sleep problems, digestive health and detoxification are the most commonly overlooked aspects of a hormonal health program. The digestive, endocrine and nervous systems are the three interrelated systems that control all hormones in the body. So remember, anything that upsets your digestion also has the potential to throw your hormones way out of whack.

The hormones produced in your digestive tract not only govern appetite, food breakdown, nutrient absorption and waste excretion, but also influence your mood, mind and memory. These chemicals are secreted in the gastrointestinal (GI) tract, especially in the stomach and small intestine. They are released in response to your food intake, as well as stretching of the digestive tract wall, stress and many other factors. Once released into the bloodstream, these compounds affect other areas outside the digestive tract, including the brain, liver, pancreas and fat cells. In other words, a single hormone can ultimately influence many different bodily functions besides digestion, including appetite, cognition and mood, growth, fertility and metabolism.

The foods you choose and the function of your digestive tract both strongly influence your nervous system and your endocrine system. Their effects can in turn alter your hormones, inflammatory response and you guessed it—impact your weight-loss success by hampering your ability to burn fat, control appetite or curb cravings.

Some digestive problems are caused or exacerbated by adverse reactions to particular foods. Such reactions can impair the release of enzymes and the movement of food through your intestines and the walls of your GI tract. An extreme example is celiac disease, an allergic reaction to gluten (commonly found in wheat, rye, barley, malt and select grains) that interferes with nutrient absorption. In other cases, the barrier of the intestinal wall can become permeable, allowing foreign substances to pass into the bloodstream. When this disruption occurs, inflammation, immune compromise or allergies may follow and lead to hormonal imbalance.

In order to function at its healthy best, your digestive system needs:

- Relief from inflammation, food allergies and poor food choices
- Release from the grip of stress and tension

- The right bacterial balance for immunity and for ridding the body of excess estrogen
- Proper enzymes and acid levels for nutrient absorption
- Open communication with the nervous system and the brain to control appetite, metabolism and digestive functions
- The ability to "keep things moving" so it can rid the body of hormonal waste, fat and toxins

Recall that good digestion (enhanced through detoxification) offers many benefits for your overall health and well-being:
- Optimal nutrient absorption
- Effective elimination of waste
- Healthy immunity
- Healthy mind, mood and memory
- Glowing skin
- Appetite control
- Protection from the harmful effects of stress

These are just a few of the benefits you can expect to enjoy within days of beginning your Detox Diet.

HORMONE DISRUPTORS IN YOUR BEDROOM

THE TOP 10 HABITS THAT SABOTAGE YOUR SLEEP AND INTERFERE WITH FAT LOSS—AND THE RULES YOU CAN USE TO AVOID THEM

As we discussed in Chapter 2, poor sleep can wreak havoc on your hormones and impair your ability to lose fat. The following list highlights sleep-disrupting habits that can sabotage your slumber. Take a look at these offenders, and make sure you do the opposite, noted *alongside*, to optimize your sleep.

1. Eating too close to bedtime; *stop eating 3 hours before bed.*
   Late-night meals and snacks prevent your body from cooling down during sleep and raise your insulin level. As a

result, less cell-boosting melatonin and growth hormone are released while you snooze.

2. Sleeping with light exposure or too close to your digital alarm clock; *sleep in pitch dark and keep electrical equipment at least 3 feet away.*

   Even a small amount of light interferes with the release of melatonin and, subsequently, the release of growth hormone. Cortisol also remains abnormally high when you are exposed to light. You should also be aware of electromagnetic fields (EMFs) that are emitted from electrical devices and digital alarm clocks in your bedroom. These can disrupt the pineal gland and the production of melatonin and serotonin. Research has also linked EMFs to increased risk of cancer. If you must use these items, try to keep them as far away from the bed as possible—at least 3 feet away—and turn the light display away from your line of sight.

3. Too much liquid before bed; *stop drinking 2 hours before bedtime and use a red night light in the bathroom, if a night light is needed.*

   Drinking before bedtime can definitely increase your need for late-night trips to the toilet. Waking to go to the bathroom interrupts your natural sleep patterns. If you turn the light on when you go, you also run the risk of suppressing melatonin production.

4. Exercising late at night; *avoid cardiovascular exercise in the 3-hour period before bed.*

   Regular exercise can certainly help you sleep better, as long as you do it early enough in the day. A late-night workout, especially a cardio session, raises body temperature significantly, preventing the release of melatonin. It can also interfere with your ability to fall asleep, since it usually increases noradrenaline, dopamine and cortisol, which stimulate brain activity.

5. Too much TV or computer use before bed; *take time to "power down" and focus on mind-calming activities.*

   Many of us enjoy watching favorite TV shows, catching up on emails or surfing the Net in the evenings, but too much time in front of either screen close to bedtime can interfere with a good night's rest. Both these activities increase the stimulating hormones noradrenaline and dopamine, which can hamper your ability to fall asleep. Instead, opt for activities that allow you to focus on one thing like meditation, reading or journaling. These habits make you serotonin dominant and improve your sleep.

6. Keeping your bedroom too warm (higher than 70°F); *sleep in a cool environment.*

   Plenty of people like to feel cozy at bedtime, but a sleep environment that's too warm can prevent the natural cooling that should take place in your body while you sleep. Without this cool-down process, melatonin and growth hormone release is disrupted, which means you won't burn fat while you sleep or benefit from nighttime repair of your bones, skin and muscles.

7. Sleeping in tight-fitting clothes; *sleep in the nude and avoid excessive, heavy blankets.*

   Besides feeling comfy, your favorite PJs can actually help you sleep better, but not if they're too tight. Wearing tight-fitting clothing at bedtime—even a bra or underwear—appears to raise your body temperature and has been proven to reduce the secretion of melatonin and growth hormone. Your best bet is to sleep in the nude. If you prefer to wear something to bed, make sure it's light and loose fitting.

8. Failure to open the blinds or go outside in the morning; *let the light in as soon as you wake.*

   Remember, melatonin is supposed to be lowest first thing in the morning. If you remain in darkness, your body will not get the signal that the time has come to get up and go. High melatonin during the day leaves you feeling fatigued and unable to wake up properly. It may also lower serotonin, leading to depression, anxiety and cravings.

9. **Not getting the right amount of sleep;** *aim for 7.5 to 9 hours nightly.*

    The American Cancer Association found higher incidences of cancer in individuals who consistently slept 6 hours or less or more than 9 hours nightly. New research recently reported that people who regularly sleep 7.5 hours per night live longer. Most sleep experts agree that 7 to 8 hours a night is optimal. However, some people may require more or less sleep than others. If you wake without an alarm and feel refreshed when you get up, you're likely getting the right amount of sleep for you.

    When your sleep is insufficient, your cortisol and hunger hormones both surge, causing a corresponding increase in insulin. You also experience decreases in leptin, melatonin, growth hormone, testosterone and serotonin, all of which lead to weight gain.

10. **Going to bed too late;** *hit the sack between 10 and 11 p.m. nightly.*

    More than half the respondents to the 2005 National Sleep Survey reported they are morning people with higher energy earlier in the day, while 41 percent considered themselves night owls. Evening people were more likely than morning people to experience symptoms of insomnia and sleep apnea, enjoy less sleep than they felt they needed and take longer to fall asleep.

    Staying awake into the wee hours causes hormonal imbalance because it increases cortisol, decreases leptin and depletes growth hormone. It can cause us to eat more, and it messes with our metabolism. Cortisol naturally

begins to increase during the second half of your sleep—
a small boost at 2 a.m., another at 4 a.m. and the peak at
around 6 a.m. If you're just getting to bed immediately
beforehand, you're missing out on your most restful period
of sleep. I advocate getting to bed between 10 p.m. and
11 p.m. nightly for this basic reason.

You are now armed with the information you need to detoxify
your body and get into healthy, hormone-enhancing sleep habits.
Now you are ready to focus on your nutrition habits.

The *Supercharged* Hormone Plan: Detox

*During the coming weeks, you will have two Step 1 meals a day, with 1 to
2 detox-friendly shakes daily.*

Make sure you avoid the forbidden foods (listed on page 60). Do not
miss meals and have at least one snack. If you cut your food intake too
much, you'll simply hamper your metabolism by creating (or aggravat-
ing) imbalances in your stress and blood sugar hormones. At the end
of this chapter, you will also find a summary of your prescription for
the detox step of the *Supercharged* Hormone Diet together with a complete selection of recommended foods and recipes in Part Two.

You will begin by removing all of the foods that upset your hormones, increase inflammation, cause cravings or an allergic response.
You will also consume supplements and shakes that will help to support the removal of toxins from your body. The meals for all 4 weeks
of the *Supercharged* Hormone Diet are also slightly higher in protein
than those in the original Hormone Diet to intensify your results. I
have increased the protein because it does wonderful things for your
metabolism and your hormones, including the following:

- The very act of eating stimulates your metabolism, but
  especially so when you consume protein. Known as the
  Thermic Effect of Food (TEF), this is the amount of calories

that it takes your body to digest, absorb, transport and metabolize your food. It makes up approximately 5 to 15 percent of your total daily calorie expenditure. Protein tends to increase TEF at a rate double that of carbs and almost triple that of fats, which is one of the reasons I advocate having an adequate amount of protein at each meal.

- Eating protein also helps to support muscle growth and repair, especially after your Hormone Diet workouts.
- Higher protein intake keeps your blood sugar balanced and your insulin levels low—a metabolic must for appetite control and fat loss. The recipes are also higher in protein to make up for the reduced selection of carbohydrates. Don't worry, you will be consuming enough food, and this specific ratio will allow for better hormonal balancing effects.
- Protein is a necessary building block for many hormones, including serotonin, melatonin, growth hormone, thyroid hormone and dopamine. If we fail to get enough protein in our diet, we can experience mood disorders, memory loss, increased appetite and cravings, decreased metabolism, sleep disruption, muscle loss and weight gain. In addition to helping you preserve metabolically active muscle tissue, protein may help you maintain bone density. In a study at the University of Surrey, researchers found that protein may also increase the hormone that boosts bone mineral density.
- Protein packs a hormonal punch because it stimulates the activity of many of our fat-burning and appetite-controlling hormones when we consume it in the right amounts. A higher-protein diet helps to shed stubborn belly fat, according to a study published in *Diabetes Care* (March 2002). Researchers compared a high-protein diet with a low-protein diet in 54 obese men and women with type 2 diabetes. Those on the high-protein diet had significantly greater reductions in total and abdominal fat mass and a greater reduction in LDL cholesterol.

Forbidden Foods for The Supercharged Hormone Diet
Detox Step 1

The following food groups *must be removed from your diet* during the detox because they are inflammatory or allergenic:

Dairy products: Yogurt, cheese, milk, cream, sour cream, cottage cheese, casein and whey protein concentrate are to be *avoided*. One hundred percent pure whey protein isolate, sheep's-milk and goat's-milk cheeses are *allowed*.

All grains and grain products: Stay away from wheat, spelt, rye, oats, kamut, amaranth, barley, millet, rice, buckwheat, durum semolina, quinoa, etc. Note that most breads, bagels, muffins, pastries, cakes, pasta, couscous, cookies, flour and cereals are off-limits.

Vegetables: Enjoy ultimate amounts of all vegetables, except corn. Potatoes, including sweet potatoes and white potatoes, are allowed during the second week only. All other starchy vegetables, including squash, turnip, pumpkin, beets, carrots, and peas are permitted during both week 1 and week 2.

Oils: Eliminate all hydrogenated oils, palm kernel oil, trans fatty acids, soybean oil, corn oil, cottonseed oil, vegetable oil, shortening and margarine. Limit your intake of safflower and sunflower oil. Extra-virgin olive oil is *allowed*.

Alcohol and caffeine: Too much of either one will elevate stress hormones, cause cravings and contribute to hormonal imbalance. During your detox, I recommend you cut these out completely.

Peanuts and peanut-containing products: Avoid peanut butter, peanuts in the shell, trail mix containing peanuts, etc. Check labels carefully, as many products list peanuts as ingredients. My only possible exceptions are the recommended protein bars (pages 135–36), which may contain some peanuts.

Sugars, sweeteners and artificial sweeteners: Table sugar (sucrose) and all products with sugar and artificial sweeteners added must be cut out completely. Foods to avoid include rice syrup, maple syrup, honey, agave syrup, foods/drinks containing high-fructose corn syrup, packaged foods, candies, soft drinks, juice, etc., as well as sucralose, aspartame, saccharin and all other forms of artificial sweeteners.

Citrus fruit: Remove oranges, tangerines and grapefruit from your diet. Lemons and limes are permitted.

Red meats: Eliminate pork, beef, lamb, all types of cold cuts, bacon and all types of sausages.

IS YOUR BODY SENDING YOU SIGNALS?

The following symptoms could be signals of foods intolerances/sensitivities:

DIGESTIVE:

Abdominal cramping

Bloating

Blood in the stool

Constipation

Gas

GERD (reflux)

Indigestion or heartburn

Inflammatory bowel
disease

Irritable bowel syndrome

Lactose intolerance

Loose stools

MENTAL/EMOTIONAL:

Anxiety

Depression

Food cravings

Insomnia

Irritability

GENERAL/APPEARANCE:

Arthritis (rheumatoid)

Cellulite

Dark under-eye circles

Difficulty getting out of
bed in the morning

Difficulty losing weight

Fatigue

Headaches

High blood pressure

Joint pain or stiffness

Malaise

Migraines

Puffy eyes

Water retention

Weight gain

SKIN:

Acne

Eczema

Hives

Psoriasis

(continued)

NASAL/IMMUNE SYSTEM:

Asthma

Chronic ear infections

Ear congestion

Hay fever

Itching in the ears

Itchy mouth

Postnasal drip

Runny nose

Seasonal allergies

Sinus congestion

Sneezing

Watery eyes

Permitted Foods for The Supercharged Hormone Diet Detox: Step 1

The following anti-inflammatory and immune-enhancing foods are permissible during your detox program on a daily basis. For a handy chart on foods to avoid and enjoy during your detox, see Part Two.

Vegetables: Enjoy unlimited amounts of all vegetables *except* corn. Potatoes, including sweet potatoes and white potatoes, are allowed during the second week only. All other starchy vegetables, including squash, turnip, pumpkin, beets, carrots and peas are permitted during both week 1 and week 2.

Fruits: Eat 1 to 3 servings of all fruits *except* oranges, tangerines, grapefruit, canned fruits, raisins, dates and other non-organic dried fruits.

One serving of beans: Choose from any type of beans.

Two servings (2 tablespoons each) of nuts and seeds: Eat all nuts *except* peanuts; all seeds are fine.

Fish and meat: Enjoy all poultry (chicken, turkey, duck, etc.), fish and seafood.

Two servings of dairy (1 tablespoon): Eat sheep's- or goat's-milk feta; goat cheese; small amounts of butter but no other cow's milk products.

Oils: Restrict these to canola oil, flaxseed oil, hemp oil, coconut oil, small amounts of butter and extra-virgin olive oil.

Eggs: Use both yolks and whites.

Milks: Oat, almond and soy milks are fine, but avoid those with sugar added. Almond is my preference as it is lowest in carbs.

Sweeteners: Stevia and Xylitol are allowed.

Soy products: Organic, non-GMO (genetically modified) soy products are allowed, unless you have noticed digestive upset (gas, bloating, indigestion or similar symptoms) when you have eaten these products in the past. Selections include tofu, tempeh, soy nuts, unsweetened soy milk and whole soybeans. Keep soy consumption to a maximum of 1 serving a day. If you are taking thyroid hormone, be sure to consume soy 2 to 3 hours away from your medication.

*Note that the only difference between the first and second week of your detox is the option to add **1 daily serving of gluten-free grains or potatoes.*** One serving is $^1/_2$ cup. Your gluten-free grains or potato selections can include quinoa, millet, rice and rice products, buckwheat, rice pasta, rice cakes, rice crackers, white potatoes and sweet potatoes. However, if you notice increased hunger, cravings, water retention or weight gain after the consumption of any one of these hypoallergenic carb selections, I suggest avoiding them again. Quinoa is the best option if you wish to be the most carb-conscious.

What Can You Expect to Feel?

Don't be surprised if you experience headaches, fatigue, irritability and general malaise during the first 3 to 4 days of your detox. These symptoms are a normal side effect as your body is doing a lot of house cleaning. Rest and go to bed early if you feel sluggish. Be sure to drink a full 8 cups of water daily, or try my recipe for the *Supercharged* Hormone Diet Detox Water, which contains lemon and herbs to assist your liver and add extra vitamin C to reduce detox symptoms, if necessary. You should, however, feel your energy increasing and mental focus improving by the fourth day.

If you need encouragement and motivation to keep you on track, remember this: *the more severe your detox reactions, the more you really needed it!*

The Transition from Step 1 to Step 2

During week 3, you will slowly reintroduce many of the foods you have been avoiding in the first 2 weeks. It is at this point that you will identify potential food allergies or sensitivities. (See pages 252–254.)

THE *SUPERCHARGED* HORMONE DIET DETOX WATER

- The juice of one-half to one whole fresh organic lemon
- 1-inch piece of fresh ginger, sliced (you can omit this or add more, if you wish)
- Pinch of cayenne pepper
- 4 cups of reverse-osmosis water

While this may sound like a strange brew, consider this: the spices in this mixture increase metabolism, lower insulin, support digestion and improve liver function. Capsaicin, which is the active ingredient in cayenne, may boost sympathetic nervous system activity in a way that dampens hunger and caloric intake later in the day. Related research found that capsiate, a compound found in sweet peppers, hinders fat storage, boosts weight loss and increases metabolism. Try to drink at least 8 cups per day of this flavorful formula.

KICK THE HORMONE DISRUPTORS OUT OF YOUR KITCHEN

Lurking in your kitchen are foods that can inhibit your weight-loss success in a big way. The list below covers foods you should *never* eat. In fact, I recommend you remove them from your kitchen immediately to prevent further hormonal disruption.

- Products containing artificial sweeteners (aspartame, sucralose, etc.)
- Products containing high-fructose corn syrup
- Vegetable oil, shortening, margarine, cottonseed oil; anything containing partially hydrogenated oils; products containing trans fats
- Processed and packaged foods that contain lots of preserv-

atives, loads of sodium and few nutrients, e.g., prepared pasta side dishes

The next step to remove hormone disruptors in your kitchen is to get rid of your plastic food storage containers and replace them with glass. Use paper wraps instead of plastic whenever possible; if you do use plastic wraps, make sure those you put in contact with food do not contain phthalates (if you're not sure, ask the manufacturer). Never microwave foods in plastic containers or Styrofoam, which may leach harmful compounds. Potentially harmful or cancer-causing, estrogen-like chemicals called dioxins can leach into your foods and drinks, especially when heated or frozen. Always choose metal, glass or wood instead of plastic for storing, reheating and serving foods.

We've all heard about the potential dangers of soft plastic water bottles. Avoid these as much as you can and never drink your water if it has been heated or frozen in your car. Do not refill bottles. When you need to, try to purchase water or juice products in glass bottles. You may want to consider a reverse-osmosis water system for your kitchen tap. It is much less expensive than buying a unit for the whole house.

For cooking, avoid aluminum pots and pans because usage of these materials has been associated with an increased risk of Alzheimer's disease (the same goes for antiperspirants that contain aluminum). Limiting or eliminating your exposure to Teflon-coated pans is also a good idea, as the chemical used to make the non-stick substance is currently being studied for potential health risks.

Finally, a word on cleaning products and kitchenware: choose household and laundry cleaning alternatives that are less toxic than standard products. Examples of less-toxic cleaners include Kosher Soap, Citra Solv, Borax, That Orange Stuff and Nature Clean. For your laundry, consider the non-toxic household products by Seventh Generation (seventhgeneration.com).

The Details on Good Digestion

Keeping your bowels moving regularly is critical at all times, but especially during your detox, to avoid accumulation and reabsorption of toxins from the bowels. You should be having at least one to three bowel movements per day. On occasion, dietary changes or reduced intake of fibrous grains can cause constipation, though almost all people report that the Clear Detox—Digestive Health product available at clearmedicine.com helps significantly with bowel regularity (even though they are laxative-free and cannot create a harmful dependence). Try one or more of these solutions to keep things "moving along," if you find you need some help:

- **Increase your intake of fiber.** A fiber supplement providing 8 to 10 g of fiber per serving should be used in your smoothies and detox shakes. Add 1 or 2 tablespoons of ground flaxseed or chia seed daily to your meals, salads or drinking water is also an excellent means of increasing your fiber. Whether you purchase it ground or grind your own, flaxseed should be kept in the freezer for maximum freshness. Your selection of fiber supplement should be a non-irritating, psyllium-free fiber powder or capsule such as Clear Fiber (Clear Medicine), Solufibre (AOR) or Gentle Fibers (Jarrow).

- **Increase vitamin C.** Take 3 to 8 g of vitamin C (spread out throughout the day, not all at once). Vitamin C is a natural laxative in higher doses. The absolute best vitamin C for beating constipation that I have found is Effer-C (Douglas Labs). Try $1/2$ to 1 teaspoon in water before bed.

- **Take magnesium citrate or glycinate.** This supplement can encourage bowel movements because it's a natural muscle relaxant. Take 200 to 800 mg per day. Start with a low dose and increase it gradually (as with the vitamin C, take your magnesium throughout the day). I usually recommend 200 to 600 mg at bedtime.

Ghrelin is a hormone produced in your stomach and upper intestine. This hormone stimulates appetite when your brain senses the absence of food in your belly. When you are hungry and your stomach is growling like a grizzly bear, ghrelin is being produced.

Peptide YY is an appetite inhibitor produced in the GI tract and released in response to the presence of protein. Eating protein regularly throughout the day will do wonders for keeping your appetite in check. Consuming your protein first at mealtime can also help stop you from overeating.

Cholecystokinin (CCK) causes the pancreas to produce the enzymes that break down protein, carbs and fats. It also causes your gallbladder to release bile into your small intestine. CCK is released when we eat fats. It's part of the reason that fats make us feel full and satisfied and also why low-fat diets are not sustainable. High-fiber foods also promote CCK release.

The *Supercharged* 30-Day Supplement Plan

While you are on this 30-day plan, you should also include the supplements outlined in this section. They are not a mandatory part of your program, but they will enhance your results considerably. These supplements will:

- Improve the breakdown and elimination of hormones in the liver and digestive system
- Provide additional antioxidant protection
- Boost your energy and increase your metabolic rate
- Reduce cravings

I have recommended specific brands, but don't feel you have to purchase these exact products. Products with similar ingredients should be fine, provided they are from a reputable company. You can certainly ask the staff at your local health-food store for advice. If you don't have a health-food store near you, try searching the Internet for companies that ship or visit drnatashaturner.com.

1. **A high-quality probiotic supplement**: Healthy bacterial balance in the digestive system is vital for overall health, particularly for the breakdown and elimination of estrogen. Probiotics assist with bowel cleansing, preventing constipation, reducing allergy symptoms and boosting immunity and skin health. Some studies suggest that the bacteria in your stomach can actually impact your weight-loss efforts. Researchers at Emory University found that mice bred to have an altered balance of bacteria in their intestines were 20 percent heavier after 5 months than their counterparts that weren't bred that way. Changes in concentration of some bacteria may cause inflammation, leading to an increase in appetite and insulin resistance. So perfect balance truly begins from the inside out! While yogurt naturally contains probiotics, supplements are more effective as a concentrated source. All probiotic supplements should be refrigerated. During your detox, I recommend a probiotic with at least 10 to 15 billion cells per capsule, such as Clear Flora, while a good maintenance dose is 1 to 2 billion of both lactobacilli and bifidobacteria once a day, away from food.

   Some people experience bloating when they first begin taking probiotic supplements. If you are bothered by this effect, simply reduce the dosage and slowly increase it again as your body adapts.

   Recommended brands include:
   - **Clear Flora (Clear Medicine)**: 2 capsules on rising
   - **Multi-Probiotic 4000 (Douglas Labs)**: 2 capsules on rising
   - **Bio-K+**: 1 jar (away from food) or 1 capsule per day (with food)
   - **Smooth Food 2** or **Probiotic All-Flora (New Chapter)**: 2 capsules per day

   Note: These products must be refrigerated.

2. **An herbal cleansing formula for the liver and/or bowels that contains milk thistle, dandelion, turmeric, artichoke and/or beet leaf:** These herbs improve the flow of bile, aid liver function, reduce inflammation, improve estrogen and cortisol metabolism and reduce fatty liver, a factor known to accelerate aging and weight gain.

   Recommended brands include:
   - **Clear Detox—Hormonal Health (Clear Medicine):** 1 pack per day on rising or with breakfast. This product contains not only nutrients to support liver detoxification but also ingredients to support the breakdown and elimination of harmful estrogen.
   - **L-Trepein (Thorne):** 2 capsules with breakfast and dinner.
   - **Lipogen (Metagenics):** 2 capsules three times daily with meals.
   - **Liver–G.I. Detox (Pure Encapsulations):** 1 to 2 capsules with breakfast and dinner.

3. **One serving per day of a bowel-cleansing formula containing fiber:** Choices include psyllium, apple, beet or flax fibers, glutamine, the herb triphala and preferably herbs to coat and heal the digestive tract wall, such as deglycyrrhizinated licorice (DGL), aloe and/or marshmallow. This type of product will promote healthier, more frequent bowel movements while you detox your liver and digestive system. It will also help maintain the integrity of your digestive tract wall, thereby reducing inflammation and leaky gut syndrome, two causes of toxic fat gain.

   Triphala is a standardized blend of three fruit extracts—*Terminalia chebula, Terminalia belerica* and *Emblica officinalis*—in equal proportions. It is an Ayurvedic herbal blend commonly used for supporting intestinal detoxification, occasional constipation and overall colon health.

   Soluble fiber is fermented in your large intestines by your intestinal microflora and will help create an intestinal environment that allows beneficial bacteria to thrive. When taken with appropriate amounts of water, soluble fiber also bulks up the stool to support larger, softer stools and healthy bowel movements. As the bulk moves through your intestine, it helps to collect and eliminate other waste and toxins from your intestinal walls.

Recommended brands include:

- **Clear Detox—Digestive Health (Clear Medicine)**: 1 pack per day at bedtime or dinner, with a full glass of water.
- **G.I. Fortify (Pure Encapsulations)**: 1 serving per day.

Your complete 4-week *Supercharged* Hormone Diet kit can be ordered through drnatashaturner.com. The kit contains pH paper, Clear Detox—Hormonal Health, Clear Detox—Digestive Health, Clear Flora and Clear Omega ultra pure extra-strength fish oil capsules. Protein powder and bars can also be added to your order and can help beat cravings. Clear Fiber, with 7 grams of fiber, is also available at this website.

4. **A daily dose of sunshine and a vitamin D3 supplement:**
Vitamin D has been proven to lower insulin, improve serotonin levels, enhance the immune system and even improve fat-loss efforts. A study conducted at University of Minnesota found higher vitamin D levels in the body at the start of a low-calorie diet improved weight-loss success. The researchers determined that for every slight increase in the level of vitamin D3, subjects ended up losing almost a half pound extra. Moreover, higher baseline vitamin D levels predicted greater loss of abdominal fat. Take 2,000 to 5,000 IU daily for optimal results and long-term health.

**BOOT THE HORMONE DISRUPTORS
OUT OF YOUR BATHROOM:**

Think of all the products we put on our skin and imagine how the daily absorption of these chemicals adds up over a lifetime. This long-term exposure is a definite hormonal and health concern. I want you to use this list to help you to avoid harmful chemicals in your cosmetics and skin care. Some ingredients are not only hormone disruptors, but also listed by the US Environmental Protection Agency and the State of California as a carcinogen risk:

1. Acrylamide
2. Ethylene oxide
3. Formaldehyde
4. Phthalates

Your cleansing products should be free of sodium lauryl sulfate, a harsh detergent present in shampoos and cleansers. The products you use on your body or face should be free of methyl parabens, propyl parabens, formaldehyde, imidazolidinyl urea, methylisothiazolinone, propylene glycol, paraffin, isopropyl alcohol and sodium lauryl sulfate. You should know that most perfumed products contain many of these harmful chemicals, but the ingredients are not identified on the label. Therefore, look for products that contain natural oils and fragrances. Here are my favorite brands for natural skin care products:

- **Korres**—The company makes amazing body butters, lip balms, body lotions.
- **Naturopathica**—I love their Environmental Defense Mask.
- **Juice Beauty**—The Green Apple Peel is a fabulous exfoliant.
- **Burt's Bees**—They make a wonderful array of products for the whole family.
- **SkinCeuticals**—I love their hyaluronic acid serum and vitamin C serum.
- **John Masters**—I adore the green tea and vitamin C facial serums, blood orange body moisturizer and all of their shampoos and conditioners.
- As a natural alternative to perfume, use body oils that are scented with natural essential oils.

Taming Tummy Troubles: Personalizing Your Nutrition and Supplements

As I noted earlier, we must solve digestive woes while your body works to rid itself of toxic buildup. In this next section, I list many of the common digestive problems and natural ways to get relief that are free of side effects.

GAS AND BLOATING

If you find that you have persistent gas and bloating, even after the removal of potential trigger foods and the addition of a probiotic for at least 5 days, then taking a digestive enzyme with meals is the next logical step. Look for one that contains a mixture of enzymes for breaking down protein, carbohydrates and fats (proteases, amylases and lipases, respectively). My favorites are Ultrazyme from Douglas Labs, Digestive Enzymes Ultra from Pure Encapsulations, or Digest Plus from Genestra. Udo's Enzymes are also a valuable option available at most health-food stores.

HEARTBURN, INDIGESTION OR ACID REFLUX

Unfortunately, people with *reduced* acid levels frequently suffer from what they assume are symptoms of elevated stomach acid, including heartburn, bloating, nausea and frequent burping. As a result, they reach for over-the-counter acid-reducing remedies, which can actually encourage greater imbalance and increase the risk of developing peptic or duodenal ulcers and even pancreatic or gastric cancer. These drugs also reduce our nutrient-absorption capabilities, which can have far-reaching negative effects. For example, vitamin B12 is crucial for heart health because of its ability to reduce homocysteine.

Antacids reduce stomach acid. Stomach acid is essential for the absorption of vitamin B12. So, when you take antacids, you can become at risk of vitamin B12 deficiency.

Choose all supplements and medications carefully, and always investigate their potential side effects—sometimes beyond what you see on the label. Natural supplements work wonderfully to help with indigestion and heartburn. Believe it or not, excess acidity in the stomach is much less common and is usually not the cause of your discomfort. Consider all options for treating low acidity, such as the HCl challenge, which will help you to determine if low acidity is a concern. The instructions for this challenge are in the Book Extras section of the book at drnatashaturner.com. Remember to take a peek at your fingernails too. Vertical ridges can indicate poor nutrient absorption related to low stomach HCl.

Natural products can often effectively reduce the symptoms of heartburn, indigestion or reflux without the risk of further decreasing stomach acid. Consider:

- DGL—Take a 500 mg capsule before or after meals.
- Slippery elm, marshmallow and/or plantain—These herbs are called demulcents; they coat and heal your digestive tract wall. Many herbal companies make remedies containing a blend of these. Try Heartburn Essentials (Pure Encapsulations). Take 2 capsules on rising and before bed for at least 3 to 4 months.
- Aloe vera—Try adding 2 to 4 ounces to your daily protein shakes.
- Liquid calcium magnesium—Take 1 tablespoon after meals and/or before bed.
- Fennel, anise or chamomile—Take in a tea or tincture form to ease the discomfort of gas or bloating.
- Digestive enzymes may reduce reflux symptoms caused by low stomach acid levels.

In addition to any of the above healing herbs, taking glutamine can help heal the digestive tract lining. Regardless of the remedy you choose, I recommend you continue treatment well after the symptoms of heartburn or reflux have subsided—at least 3 to 4 months for complete restoration of healthy cells in the digestive tract wall.

Helicobacter pylori is a type of bacterium that tends to overgrow when our stomach acidity is low. Overgrowth of *H. pylori* also tends to cause a reduction in stomach acidity, thereby allowing *H. pylori* to proliferate. This nasty infiltration increases the likelihood of colonization of the stomach and small intestine by other unwelcome organisms as well. The end result is heartburn, gastritis, duodenal ulcer or gastric ulcer. *H. pylori* infections can also lead to some forms of arthritis (calcification, spurs), iron deficiency, anemia and vitamin B12 deficiency. *H. pylori* is even associated with heart disease, gum disease, rosacea, asthma and chronic headaches or migraines.

If you have frequent heartburn, esophageal irritation or reflux you should ask your doctor to order a test for an overgrowth of *H. pylori*. Proper treatment of *H. pylori* is critical, as new research has found that high levels of this bacterium may be linked to certain cancers of the digestive tract.

Natural treatment options for *H. pylori* overgrowth:

- Mastica gum is a wonderful natural agent to restore healthy bacterial balance and heal the digestive tract.
- Berberine is a natural antibiotic, good for treating traveller's diarrhea as well as *H. pylori*. Look for products such as Candibactin-BR from Metagenics, Enterocap from Thorne Research or Anti-MFP from Douglas Labs.
- Oregano oil is helpful in either a capsule or drop form.
- Hydrochloric acid supplements should be taken with each meal to suppress the growth of *H. pylori*.
- Digestive enzymes (including pancreatic enzymes, plant-based enzymes, papaya, bromelain or pepsin) should be taken with each meal to aid nutrient absorption.
- Test your B12 levels. Optimal values are greater than 600 in the blood.

Treatment should continue for 8 weeks. Tests for *H. pylori* levels should be completed both before and after treatment. You may require additional treatment with antibiotics if your levels still do not return to normal. Be sure to follow all antibiotics with a high potency probiotic supplement to keep yeast growth under control.

YEAST OVERGROWTH OR CHRONIC YEAST INFECTIONS

Like *H. pylori* bacterium, *Candida albicans* yeast occurs naturally in the digestive tract and tends to overgrow in a pH-imbalanced environment. Yeast in the digestive tract is also controlled by our friendly bacterium, *Lactobacillus acidophilus*. If you have ever experienced a yeast infection after a course of antibiotics, now you know why.

Antibiotics can disrupt our healthy bacterial balance by killing off our beneficial bacteria together with the "bad," infection-causing bacteria, leaving a perfect environment for yeast to grow and flourish. When yeast growth gets out of hand, a yeast infection in the mouth (thrush) or genitals can result. Yeast infections may also be caused by the birth control pill, immune compromise (which allows opportunistic infections such as candidiasis to occur), immune-suppressing steroid medications, parasitic infections, diabetes and consumption of excess carbohydrates, sugar or alcohol.

Either type of yeast infection can spread to other parts of the body, resulting in less obvious but chronic symptoms, including:

1. Constipation, diarrhea
2. Gas, bloating or belching, especially after consuming fruit, sugar, alcohol or fermented products such as vinegars
3. Chronic nasal congestion or sinus problems
4. Rectal itching
5. Recurrent urinary tract infections
6. Recurrent vaginal yeast infections
7. Fatigue

Depression, irritability, difficulty concentrating, headaches and dizziness may also arise because of the production of by-products of yeast in the digestive tract, which enter the circulation through the digestive tract wall to ultimately affect the brain and nervous system.

If you are experiencing some of these symptoms and suspect they may be connected to chronic yeast overgrowth, you may wish to add antiyeast treatments to your detox. But an important first step in treating candidiasis is to ensure that you do indeed have a yeast infection. Misdiagnosis is common, and studies have shown that as many as two-thirds of all over-the-counter drugs sold for yeast infections are used by women without the condition. Using these drugs when they are not needed may lead to a resistant infection, which becomes much more difficult to treat.

Opting for over-the-counter or prescription treatments for yeast infections, when indicated, may provide symptomatic relief, but many are ineffective for chronic or recurring infections. The following tips can help you attack the source of the problem and find a lasting cure.

Change your diet. Yeast feed on sugar, vinegar, fungus and fermented foods. If you cut off their food supply, the yeast will die. During the 4 weeks you will already be staying away from processed foods, including anything that contains refined sugar, white flour, white rice and alcohol, but you should also avoid anything that contains yeast and all fermented foods. Mushrooms and vinegars should also be avoided. Instead, use lemon juice as the base of your dressings. Remember, the stricter you are with your dietary changes, the less time you will have to wait before you see favorable results. Cheating will allow that pesky yeast to grow again!

Restore healthy bacteria. A probiotic supplement is essential during any detox, but replenishing acidophilus levels will also help to counteract an overgrowth of candida. If you need to take a prescription antibiotic to fight an infection, be sure to follow it with acidophilus supplements for twice the length of time you took the antibiotics. For maximum results, take acidophilus on an empty stomach, when you wake up or before bed. I recommend Clear Flora, a high-potency probiotic supplement that contains 15 billion cells per capsule.

Add yeast-busting antifungal agents to your detox supplement regimen. There are different strains of yeast, which means that not all cases of candidiasis will respond to the same treatment. Begin using one or two products and switch to another if you do not see improvement. Continue treatment for 4 weeks to 6 months, depending on the severity of your symptoms. Natural products to choose from include:

- Dida is a natural product designed to inhibit the overgrowth of yeast. It contains antifungal (cinnamon, garlic, olive leaves and oregano) and antiseptic herbs (thyme and marigold). Peppermint and fennel are also mixed in to calm your digestive system. Take 2 tablets a day between meals for 6 weeks (see newnordic.com).
- Garlic is a great natural antifungal. It's usually taken at 4,000 to 6,000 mcg of allicin (the active ingredient in garlic) 1 to 2 times a day.
- Oregano oil is an antifungal agent that kills candida. Take it as directed on the label. It's available in both capsule and liquid form.
- Olive leaf extract is an antiviral, antibacterial and antifungal product useful for yeast infections. Typical dosage is 500 mg three times a day.
- Grapefruit seed extract is another effective antifungal agent. Take 50 to 200 mg one to two times daily.
- Berberine, a herbal extract, is a strong antifungal and antibacterial agent.

If all else fails, Nystatin, which has very few side effects, is available through your doctor.

The *Supercharged* Hormone Diet—Putting It All Together: A Summary of Your Complete Nutrition and Supplement Prescription for 4 Weeks

WEEK OF PROGRAM	30-DAY SUPPLEMENT PRESCRIPTION	WEEKLY PROGESSION OF THE NUTRITION PRESCRIPTION
Step 1 (Week 1)	Focus: Removal of Toxic Estrogen, Liver Detox and Digestive Support 1. Clear Detox—Hormonal Health—1 pack before breakfast or lunch 2. Clear Detox—Digestive Health—1 pack at bedtime	HD Detox program, including no grains or potatoes
Detox— Step 1 (Week 2)	3. Probiotic Supplement such as Clear Flora—take 2 capsules on rising 4. pH paper to test your urine and saliva pH levels	HD Detox with the optional addition of 1 serving of gluten-free grains or potatoes daily
Transition Phase (Week 3)	5. Vitamin D3—2000 IU to 5000 IU pills with a meal daily Optional addition—highly recommended: 1. A high-potency fish oil supplement like Clear Omega—take 2 capsules with breakfast and dinner	Transition from HD Detox toward the Glyci-Med approach via the introduction of one new food each day to identify food sensitivities
Step 2— Hormonally Balanced Nutrition (Week 4)	Optional addition—specific supplements for digestive symptom relief presented in this chapter Optional addition—sleep/stress support (see Chapter 10 for options)	Glyci-Med Approach

"A totally integrated program, Dr. Turner's *The Hormone Diet* presents valuable information and detailed action plans geared to optimum food, nutrition and exercise programs. Look no longer—this program is for life, and I am thrilled with my newly gained knowledge and weight loss!"

MAURA

STATS	JAN	FEB	LOST
Weight	242	220.8	21.2
Fat Mass	103.3	91.4	11.9
Body Fat	42%	35%	7%
BP	130/90	119/77	↓
Waist (inches)	50.25	47	3.25
Hips (inches)	52	47.5	4.5

INITIAL CHIEF COMPLAINTS:

1. Obesity
2. Joint pain
3. Stamina/physical dexterity
4. Poor digestion
5. Cravings

CHAPTER 5:

THE *SUPERCHARGED* EXERCISE PRESCRIPTION

A man too busy to take care of his health is
like a mechanic too busy to take care of his tools.

SPANISH PROVERB

If you read or completed *The Hormone Diet,* my first book, you might recall that I didn't recommend or stress the importance of exercise until the fourth week of my plan. This was simply because I wanted you first to focus on optimizing your sleep, detoxifying your body and optimizing your nutrition. But this is the *Supercharged* Hormone Diet, which means more quickly beginning all of the habits and activities that will bring you great results.

During the next 4 weeks, we want your nervous system to recuperate from stress, to activate muscle function and prevent the stress of overexercising. Keep in mind that whether you engage in strength training or aerobic activity, cortisol is released during exercise in proportion to the intensity of effort. Both high-intensity and prolonged exercise cause increases in cortisol, which can remain elevated for several hours following a vigorous workout. Numerous studies have proven that this rise in cortisol tends to occur with very strenuous exercise and when we exercise for longer than 40 to 45 minutes. Repeated strenuous workouts without appropriate rest between sessions can also result in chronically elevated cortisol.

We know that chronically high cortisol can cause muscle breakdown, suppress our immune function and contribute to stubborn abdominal fat. Researchers at the University of North Carolina have also linked strenuous, fatiguing exercise to higher cortisol and lower thyroid hormones. Remember, thyroid hormones stimulate your metabolism, so depletion is definitely not a desired effect of exercise! The same study found thyroid hormones remained suppressed, even 24 hours after recovery, while cortisol levels remained high throughout the same period.

Overexercising can lead to loss of muscle, frequent colds and flus, stress, an increase in free radicals, poor recovery after exercise and slower gains from your workout efforts. Plus, your risk of illness and injury increases as your metabolic rate slows. Certainly these are not the effects you were looking for when you joined the gym. If you are a gym bunny, don't worry about taking some time off from your rigorous workout routine at this point in your program to avoid placing undue stress on your body. In fact, you can take weeks off from the gym without losing strength, according to research from Japan. In the study, people followed an exercise program for 3 months and then took a 3-month break. At the end of their hiatus, they were just as strong as they had been before taking time off. So starting your program with yoga and walking will provide the perfect amount of movement to wake up your metabolism without causing excess strain on your body.

Youthful Yoga

With its full spectrum of poses, yoga can bring the body back into its natural alignment, level out muscular imbalances and improve physical weaknesses. If you are an athlete, yoga can improve your performance by enhancing your flexibility, relaxation, breathing and balance. Anyone can improve posture, energy and endurance with regular yoga practice. Yoga offers fabulous benefits for calming your nervous system, restoring hormonal balance *and* strengthening your muscles.

Yoga is a terrific stress reliever. Numerous studies, including one completed in 2003 by the Center for Integrative Medicine of Thomas

(continued on page 84)

SIX UNDENIABLE REASONS
WHY YOU SHOULD MEDITATE

We've all been there—your day is so busy and your to-do list so long that even bathroom breaks are strategically slotted in. Between running my own business, traveling, writing, speaking engagements and media tours, my schedule can get pretty hectic. But I'll let you in on my little sanity saver: meditation. And I'm not talking about hours each day. I do 10 minutes at the start of my day, and the odd class when I can fit it in. Read on for the healthy reasons I get in my daily reflection and how it can help you too.

IT HELPS YOU BE MORE COMPASSIONATE. While it won't bring world peace, it may get us closer to it. A team of researchers from Northeastern and Harvard universities examined the effects meditation would have on compassion and virtuous behavior, and results were highly in favor of this little Zen habit. The study found that those who meditated for 8 weeks were more compassionate to a test subject and more likely to assist a stranger in need. While I can't think of anyone who wouldn't benefit from this, it's particularly helpful if you're in a field where you're coaching individuals toward better health, success and well-being (from a nutritionist to a personal trainer to a health practitioner).

IT CAN HELP YOU PERFORM BETTER ON TESTS. I have a few rituals that I engage in before a media interview, from taking phosphatidylcholine (it increases concentration) to vocal preparation to wearing a certain color underwear (true story). Add to that, a few moments of meditation to boost mental clarity and focus, often when I'm sitting in the green room or immediately upon wakening. One study, from George Mason University, found that students who followed basic meditation instructions before a lecture scored better on a quiz than their Zen-free counterparts. "The data from this study suggests that meditation may help students who might have trouble paying attention or focusing," says

Robert Youmans, the study's lead researcher and an assistant professor of psychology.

IT WILL BOOST YOUR CREATIVITY. I would love to say that while I was writing my books I never experienced writer's block, but that wouldn't be accurate. In fact, my last two books, *The Carb Sensitivity Program* and *The Supercharged Hormone Diet* had extremely tight deadlines (2 to 3 months from start to finish). When I had more ideas in my mind than what was coming out of the keyboard, I often took time to get silent and meditate. Researchers from Leiden University discovered that different types of meditation can have a profound effect on two main components of creativity: divergent thinking (which gives birth to ideas) and convergent thinking (which is more solution-focused). The key is to determine what works for you and gets you in that creative space.

IT KEEPS YOUR BLOOD PRESSURE IN CHECK. One trick to meditating is to focus on the sound of your breathing and how it feels flowing in and out of the edge of your nostrils. I find it useful to imagine my breath washing in and out like waves on the beach. You can also pick a word or a phrase that's soothing or meaningful to you. One patient of mine, an extremely tense 85-year-old man with high blood pressure, picked the word quiet, which I thought was a great choice. Repeat the word or phrase to yourself each time you exhale. As an added benefit—that patient eventually got off his blood pressure medication. According to a paper published in the journal, *Hypertension,* meditation can help patients with high blood pressure, particularly if they don't tolerate standard medications.

IT RELIEVES YOUR ACHES AND PAINS. I've written a lot about inflammation and how it affects not just your joints, but your weight, digestion, immune system and more. According to neuroscientists from the University of Wisconsin–Madison, meditation is particularly beneficial for people suffering from chronic inflammatory conditions, such as rheumatoid arthritis, inflammatory bowel disease and asthma. I can't count the number of times I've seen massive breakthroughs in my patients by taking 20 minutes a day to follow a guided or solo meditation (together with nutrition and lifestyle changes). I once had a patient swear that it helped her stop drinking and restore her confidence after years of battling with alcoholism, depression and chronic pain. You know how your aches and pains seem to vanish while on vacation, sipping an iced tea and listening to the ocean? That's meditation.

IT INCREASES AWARENESS. I've always found that the more body aware I am, the better I can recognize shifts in my own hormones and I strongly encourage my patients to do the same. This is one of many essential lessons that meditation can teach you. During a session, it's important to practice body awareness and check for tension, especially in your jaw, scalp, forehead, shoulders, lower back and hips by consciously examining each body part. Relax the areas that feel tight, as you continue breathing. This very practice (and, ideally, habit) will enable you to recognize the signs of stress during the day so you can catch yourself and keep your cortisol under wraps. It's no surprise that this mindfulness has been shown to empower people to better respond to physical cues of hunger and fullness as well.

Jefferson University in collaboration with the Yoga Research Society, have shown that yoga can lower blood cortisol levels in healthy men and women. It also is known to reduce adrenaline and stimulate the calming brain chemical GABA. Research from Boston University School of Medicine and McLean Hospital published in the *Journal of Alternative and Complementary Medicine* (May 2007) suggests yoga should be explored as a possible treatment for disorders often associated with low GABA levels, such as depression and anxiety. However, its benefits extend even further: a study conducted by Ohio State University and published in *Psychosomatic Medicine* (January 2010) indicates that yoga may act to reduce inflammation in the body. In this research, 50 subjects were divided into 2 groups: those who regularly participated in yoga and a group of yoga beginners. Researchers assessed blood samples from each of the subjects and found that those in the novice group had 41 percent higher levels of an inflammatory compound called interleukin-6 versus their more advanced peers.

If you struggle with excess belly fat or sleep disruption, yoga is a stellar choice of workout. It's also excellent if you have fertility concerns. For all these reasons, it is included in your supercharged 4-week plan. I want you to try to practice yoga twice a week for the next 4 weeks. You can purchase a yoga DVD or look for a yoga studio in your area. There are many types of yoga; my favorites are ashtanga, Anusara or hatha, but find the practice that suits you best. Ashtanga is often called power yoga, while hatha is a less intense workout. Anusara is my personal favorite because I feel it falls nicely between the two.

Conservative Cardio

While high-intensity workouts should be avoided at the beginning of your detox, we want to get you moving during these 4 weeks so that your body will be primed to begin strength training, which will be your secret to lasting metabolic power. Plus, even a short stroll can be a great way to avoid cheating. Studies prove that walking after an unhealthy meal can curb the effects of stress by reducing the amounts of fatty acids, sugars and stress hormones that are released into the bloodstream and subsequently stored as fat. This gentle form of exercise strengthens nearly every aspect of your body, promotes energy during the day, encourages a relaxation response and improves the quality of your sleep.

Your light cardio prescription for the next 4 weeks is 30 minutes, done four times a week. It could include the following:

- A bike ride
- Walking on a treadmill on an incline (for a more effective workout, don't hold onto the rails)

- A power walk
- Any other cardio machine at your gym including the elliptical or exercise bike (avoid high-intensity cardio such as Spinning)

Summary: Your *Supercharged* Exercise Prescription

WEEK OF PROGRAM	WEEKLY EXERCISE PRESCRIPTION
Weeks 1, 2 and 3	2 yoga (at home with a DVD or at a class) 4 moderate cardio (30 minutes maximum)

HORMONE DIET SUCCESS STORY: ROSE

"I feel blessed to find *The Hormone Diet* to address all of my health needs. In fact, my husband decided to do the program with me, and we have both lost about 11 lbs! We no longer call it a 'program' since it's successfully changed our entire lifestyle!"

ROSE

STATS	JAN	MAR	LOST
Weight	183.2	172.4	10.8
Fat Mass	63.4	54.7	8.7
Body Fat	34%	31%	3%
BP	119/86	120/80	
Waist (inches)	37.5	35.25	2.25

INITIAL CHIEF COMPLAINTS:

1. Lack of energy
2. Mood swings
3. Trouble sleeping through the night
4. Restless, jumpy legs
5. Focus, memory problems

CHAPTER 6

STEP 2—
THE GLYCI-MED APPROACH

The entire ocean is affected by a pebble.

BLAISE PASCAL

After you have completed your body detox and identified your allergenic foods, the next area to focus on is, without a doubt, eating for glycemic balance. I came up with the Glyci-Med approach when I first wrote *The Hormone Diet*, and I'm still convinced it is the right dietary solution for lasting blood sugar and hormonal balance. This approach combines the food selections of a Mediterranean diet and the principles of glycemically balanced eating.

The Mediterranean diet is characterized by daily consumption of olive oil and an intake of monounsaturated to saturated fats that's much higher than in other parts of the world. The wonderful thing about these fats is that they help keep you full and actually encourage the loss of belly fat. In fact, eating a diet that's lower in carbs, *not* lower in fats, is the best way to lose weight. In a recent United Arab Emirates study, people who followed a low-carb diet had lower body weight, insulin levels and triglycerides than those who went with a low-fat diet. So clearly, fat-free foods don't equate to fat-free bellies!

Glycemically balanced eating simply means eating to maintain stable blood sugar, which ultimately stimulates less insulin release. Remember, the primary hormone that tells your body to store energy as fat is insulin; therefore, lower insulin is always better for fat loss. Maintaining consistent blood sugar and insulin is one of the most important steps to balancing all hormones in the body and ensuring that your metabolism stays in high gear. In fact, it's almost impossible to lose weight if your insulin levels are too high. But if you eat frequently, at the right times and consume protein, healthy fat, fiber and low glycemic carbohydrates together at every meal, you will achieve glycemic balance.

The Mediterranean diet helps protect you from many health problems, including heart disease, high blood pressure and even cancer. The Mediterranean diet is also filled with healthy fats that make your meals much healthier *and* more filling. A study conducted by researchers at the universities of Las Palmas and Navarra in Spain, published in the *Journal of the American Medical Association* (October 2009), found evidence that the Mediterranean diet may aid in the fight against depression as well. According to the researchers, those who closely adhered to the diet had a *30 percent lower* risk of developing depression.

So, with all these benefits, what could be the problem with this diet? While it helps with many areas of your health, it is *not* scientifically designed to help balance your hormones, especially insulin. So by *combining the best principles and benefits of both approaches* I have created the world's *first* diet that lets you enjoy mouth-watering, satisfying foods *and* control your blood sugar and hormones at the same time. But the total benefits of this eating style would not be possible unless we identified and reviewed your food allergies first. As a result of these combined factors, you lose weight *quickly*—and never feel hungry or food obsessed while looking and feeling your best—every day.

By following the Glyci-Med dietary approach, you will simply learn to choose the right foods at the right times and to avoid the list of foods that disrupt your hormones. Even though my recommendations seem quite basic, they are based on the most cutting-edge research for obesity treatment and prevention. Let's review the specifics:

Eat the Right Foods

- Eat lean protein, low-glycemic carbohydrates and healthy fats at each meal and snack. Following this rule will help keep your blood sugar and insulin levels stable. This means you will never eat fruit (a carb) alone. You must always have nuts or a piece of cheese (which contains fat and protein) along with it. To maintain stable blood sugar and hormones, we *must* balance our protein with carbohydrates and fats at *every* meal and snack. Taking in a steady supply of protein throughout the day is important because we can't hang onto it for later use the way we can store sugar and fat. Furthermore, essential amino acids cannot be manufactured by the body, so they *must* be a vital component of our diet.

- Avoid having a starch at breakfast most days of the week. If you stick to a high-protein breakfast, you will enjoy better appetite control and avoid that mid-afternoon slump. This means breads, cereals, bagels, etc., are off-limits. Have a protein shake or eggs instead. For your breakfast suggestions, see Part Two.

- Include olive oil (extra virgin, cold pressed), nuts, whey protein isolate and an apple in your diet each day. *You must have olive oil daily to follow the Glyci-Med approach.* Eat fresh, locally grown organic produce and choose organic or wild sources of meat, fish, eggs and dairy, which are free of hormone-disrupting additives, hormones and pesticides, whenever you can.

- For better appetite control, try having soup or salad at the beginning of your meal. Besides giving you a serving of veggies, these high-water dishes stretch your stomach and help you to feel full.

- Drink as much water as possible during the day between meals. Ideally, that means 8 to 12 cups a day for women and 16 to 20 cups a day for men. You can use the formula in The Hormone Diet Wellness Tracker in Part Three to specifically calculate your own water intake.

- Eat recommended serving sizes and avoid overeating at any one particular meal, otherwise you will create stress on your metabolism.

At the Right Times

During this week, you will begin to focus on *when* you eat. It is impossible to balance your hormones if you skip meals, eat too close to bedtime, miss your snacks or have irregular eating habits. So follow these simple timing rules:

- Aim to eat every 3 to 4 hours. Remember that the thermic effect of food can increase your metabolic rate from 5 to 15 percent after a meal, and the more small meals you eat per day, the faster your metabolism will be.
- Find the best combination of meals and snacks for you, but do not miss the afternoon meal or snack. So your option may be breakfast, snack, lunch, snack, dinner, or four equal size meals perhaps at 7 to 8 a.m., 12 to 1 p.m., 3 to 4 p.m. and 6 to 8 p.m.
- Enjoy your meals at the same time every day. People who eat at the same times daily have lower blood sugar and insulin levels, which fosters better hormonal balance for fat loss.
- Eat within 1 hour of rising and aim to avoid eating within the 3-hour period before bedtime as often as possible. Waiting too long to eat raises your cortisol and slows your metabolic rate, while eating too close to bedtime raises your body temperature and interferes with the natural fat-burning effects of sleep.
- If you are having alcohol with your meal, enjoy it *after* you eat to enhance the hormones involved in digestion and appetite control.
- If you decide to have alcohol at your meal, avoid starches (potatoes, rice, pasta, sweet potato, etc.), otherwise, you will end up consuming too much carbohydrate at one sitting.
- Always eat something within 45 minutes of finishing your workout. This meal or snack should not contain much fat and should be higher in carbohydrates with a bit of protein. This combination will maximize the release of growth hormone and stimulate muscle repair and building.

- For optimal strength and performance, never do your weight training on an empty stomach. You need adequate food to ensure you have enough energy to get through your workout effectively.
- You may complete your cardio training before eating, if your session is 30 to 40 minutes or less.

Avoid Hormone-hindering Foods

Avoid 100 percent of the time. This means you should *never* consume these products:

- Processed meats and luncheon meats. Instead, visit your local deli or butcher and ask for preservative-free (nitrate-free) sliced meats.
- Fructose-sweetened foods or foods containing high-fructose corn syrup (HFCS). HFCS increases appetite and cravings.
- Foods containing aspartame and artificial sweeteners, which raise insulin and contribute to cravings and weight gain.
- Farmed salmon. A 2004 study found higher toxin levels in farmed salmon than in wild-caught.
- Foods containing artificial coloring, preservatives, sulfites and nitrates.
- Trans fatty acids (any hydrogenated oils, partially hydrogenated oils, shortenings, margarines) and unhealthy, inflammatory fats, including most vegetable oils (sunflower, safflower), cotton seed oil and palm oil.
- Peanuts, unless they are organic and, optimally, aflatoxin-free.

Avoid 80 to 90 percent of the time. Restrict these to a maximum of 1 to 2 servings a week during your cheat meal:

- White flour, enriched flour, refined flour, wheat flour, white sugar, white potatoes, white rice.

- Saturated fats in full-fat dairy products and red meats.
- Large fish known to be high in mercury, including swordfish, shark, tilefish, marlin, orange roughy, grouper, king mackerel and tuna.
- Raisins, figs and dates because these are high in sugar and can adversely affect insulin levels.
- Choose organic chicken, turkey, pork and beef as often as you can.
- Consume coffee or caffeine as a treat (i.e., once or twice a week) rather than every day. If you feel you really can't live without it daily, choose organic coffee, stick to one cup a day and have it before lunchtime, so it will not disrupt your sleep. Decaf coffee should be avoided unless it is organic and Swiss water-processed. Your rule of coffee consumption is no sugar or sweeteners added, but a dash of cream or milk is okay, if you must have it. Add a touch of cinnamon to your coffee for a nice flavor and the sugar-regulating benefits.

What Does the Hormone Diet Plate Look Like?

At lunch and dinner, ask yourself: does my meal include carbohydrates, fat and protein? Your ideal plate should be two-thirds vegetables and one-third protein, topped with healthy fats and spices. I recommend a $^1/_2$-cup serving of starchy carbs at your evening meal to improve your sleep and serotonin balance.

Sticking with this book's philosophy of keeping things simple, a summary of the nutritional process of your *Supercharged* plan and suggested serving sizes is presented on pages 270–79. I have also outlined your carbohydrates (C), protein (P) and fat (F) selections along with your 7-day meal plan and recipes. Following the discussion of the Hot Hormone Foods in Chapter 7, Chapter 8 explains how to shop. These tools will make it easy for you to achieve total hormonal balance through a hormonally balanced diet.

More Simple Tips for Glyci-Med Balanced Meals

In addition to selecting the right types of protein, carbohydrates and fats, you can lower the glycemic impact or blood sugar impact (*and subsequently limit insulin release*) of a meal or snack using a few simple methods. Take a look at these beneficial food combinations, food prep tips and alternative food choices to improve the glycemic load of any meal or snack:

> **THE HORMONAL BENEFITS OF CARBOHYDRATES**
>
> Carbs aren't all bad! They provide us with an essential source of fiber, and they also maintain our mood by boosting serotonin. When we eliminate all carbohydrates, we raise cortisol, which increases our risk of losing metabolically active muscle.

- Studies show that having tomato juice, lemon juice or apple cider vinegar with your meal may help reduce the glycemic load.
- Choose slow-cooked oatmeal over quick oats because it is higher in fiber.
- If you really want to have a piece of pie or cake, have protein with it. Adding whey protein powder or cottage cheese will slow the release of sugars into the bloodstream and help keep insulin levels from shooting through the roof. But remember, calories in must stay below calories out for you to lose fat. Adding protein will not negate excess calories!
- Cook your pasta and rice *al dente* (firm) to maintain a moderate glycemic load. Overcooking pasta or rice raises the glycemic load.
- Lightly steam your vegetables or eat them raw to maintain their fiber content.
- Choose firm fruits that are not overly ripe. The riper the fruit, the higher the amount of naturally occurring sugars.
- If you enjoy sushi, choose sashimi instead to avoid the high glycemic load of the rice.
- Instead of a sandwich, have a salad with a scoop of sandwich filling such as egg, tuna or salmon. Two slices of bread or a bagel will raise the glycemic load of your meal.

HORMONAL HEALTH TIP

- If you crave pizza, choose a whole-wheat thin crust instead of a thick, white-flour crust. Also, always ask for extra pizza sauce to benefit from the healthy antioxidants in cooked tomatoes.
- Soups made of lentils and other legumes are better choices than, say, cream of potato because of the higher fiber content and lower glycemic value of beans versus potatoes. If your soup has a high glycemic load, consider adding low-fat cheese to increase the fat and protein content of your meal.
- If you must eat breakfast cereal, $^1/_3$ cup Ezekiel 4:9 cereal is a high-protein, high-fiber choice. Add a hard-boiled egg white or sprinkle on some vanilla whey protein powder to increase protein and slow the release of sugar into your bloodstream.
- Choose berries for dessert instead of pineapples or bananas because they are low glycemic and higher in both fiber and antioxidants.
- Dark chocolate (70 percent or higher) is a better choice than milk chocolate because it is lower in sugar and provides a source of health-promoting antioxidants. But remember, one small square is all you need to get those health benefits!
- Steer clear of low-fat, fruit-flavored yogurts, which are typically high in carbohydrates and contribute to insulin resistance. Instead, choose plain, low-fat yogurt and add your own fresh berries.
- If you must have a sweetened yogurt, choose one that is free of artificial sweeteners and mix it with some plain yogurt. The mixture will still give you the flavor you like but without as much sugar.
- The best type of bread to use is Ezekiel bread, made with sprouted grain instead of flour. Do your best to avoid white flours and white breads 80 to 90 percent of the time. If you cannot find Ezekiel, look for 100 percent whole-grain rye bread with 18 g of carbohydrate or less per slice.

94 | THE *SUPERCHARGED* HORMONE DIET

(Dimpflmeier and Stonemill breads are examples of good choices.) Use butter, almond butter, olive spreads, pesto or hummus instead of jams and jellies, which are high in sugar.

- Have whole fruits and vegetables rather than juices, which have much of the fiber removed.
- Avoid high-sugar condiments such as ketchup; choose salsa or mustard instead.
- If you do have an alcoholic drink with your dinner, skip starches such as bread, potatoes, rice or pasta. Instead, stick with lean protein and vegetables.

THE HORMONAL BENEFITS OF FIBER

Fiber offers wonderful benefits for your hormonal balance. It reduces insulin, inflammation and excess toxic estrogen. There are two types of fiber. We require both in equal amounts in our diets daily:

SOLUBLE FIBER is fantastic for lowering LDL cholesterol, and stabilizing blood sugars and insulin. Soluble fiber keeps the bowels moving and can help prevent constipation (defined as fewer than one bowel movement a day). Good sources include fruits (especially apples, pears, bananas and oranges), vegetables (broccoli, sweet potatoes, cabbage, potatoes and carrots), oat bran, barley, seed husks, flaxseed, psyllium, dried beans, lentils, peas, soy milk and other soy products.

INSOLUBLE FIBER helps to bulk up our stools, keep the bowels moving and speed up transit time of food through the digestive tract. Insoluble fiber is also your friend if you suffer from the discomfort of hemorrhoids. It's an essential part of a detox program because fiber binds to excess estrogen in the digestive tract, which is then excreted by the body. Insoluble fiber can also affect the composition of intestinal bacteria and reduce the buildup and reabsorption of free-floating estrogen. Good sources include wheat bran, corn bran, rice bran, the skins of fruits and vegetables (apples, pears, berries, tomatoes, eggplant, zucchini and carrots), nuts (especially almonds), seeds (particularly sunflower seeds), soybeans, dried beans and whole-grain foods.

You'd be surprised how hard it is to reach your intake goal of 35 to 40 g per day without a fiber supplement.

THE HORMONAL BENEFITS OF FATS

Fats prevent cravings and actually *help* us to lose weight when we consume them in the right forms and amounts. They help us feel full and satisfied because of their effects on our appetite-controlling friends, leptin and CCK.

Fats also provide "good" cholesterol, the building block of estrogen, progesterone, DHEA and cortisol.

Now that you know the rules of the Glyci-Med approach, your final 7 days of meals, a summary of foods to enjoy and foods to avoid, and more recipes are outlined for you in Part Two.

HORMONE DIET SUCCESS STORY: JANICE

"I started the Hormone Diet in January. My knee, ankle and hip joints were giving me trouble in ballet and curling. I'd been on antibiotics so many times in the past 5 years, between chronic urinary tract infections (UTIs), sinusitis and pneumonia, that I felt I needed a different approach to treating my problems. I also found that since menopause, I had little interest in sex, especially due to discomfort and fear of developing another UTI. On top of that, a nagging 15-pound weight gain over the past year really had me ticked off.

"The more entrenched I became in the Hormone Diet, the better I felt. I've learned a great deal, and I'm especially happy the program is helping eliminate the effects of all those antibiotic treatments and giving me so much more energy (and, as a big bonus, a whole lot less gas). Between that and the weekly

25-minute exercise program, I've lost 12 pounds in 2 months. The recommended supplements make so much sense and seem to be helping far more than any other treatments I've tried. And, as the inflammation is settling down, I've found I can discontinue the corticosteroid puffers and nose sprays and maintain clear lungs! I'm setting new goals and achieving more than I ever could have done on my own. I'm probably in the best shape I've been in since my early 30s when I danced full-time, but I bet I'm much healthier than I was then!"

JANICE

STATS	JAN	FEB	LOST
Weight	145.2	135.6	9.6
Fat Mass	40.9	33.5	7.4
Body Fat	28%	26%	2%
BP	124/74	106/70	↓
Waist (inches)	31	28.5	2.5
Hips (inches)	41	38.5	2.5

INITIAL CHIEF COMPLAINTS:

1. Low sex drive
2. Chronic urinary tract infections
3. Weight gain
4. Poor overall tone and core strength
5. Unhealthy aging
6. Tendonitis, arthritis

CHAPTER 7

THE HOT HORMONE FOODS

You can set yourself up to be sick, or you can choose to stay well.

WAYNE DYER

This chapter provides plenty of good news about particular foods and how you can use them to your hormonal advantage. I call them the Hot Hormone foods.

The following list gives you a snapshot of nutritious foods and drinks that help you achieve hormonal balance, feel satisfied, fight disease and lose fat. To take full advantage of all the benefits each food has to offer, follow my suggested serving guidelines. In general, though, you should enjoy all of these hormone-enhancing foods as often as you can.

Beautiful Broccoli

Broccoli and other cruciferous vegetables (cauliflower, Brussels sprouts, kale and cabbage) contain high amounts of phytonutrients called isothiocyanates, particularly two isothiocyanates called sulforaphane and indole-3-carbinol. These phytonutrients work well to increase the capacity of the liver to detoxify harmful, cancer-causing compounds. Indole-3-carbinol helps break down a harmful and potent estrogen metabolite that promotes tumor growth, especially in estrogen-sensitive breast cells. In 2008, researchers at the University of California at Berkeley showed that indole-3-carbinol halts the growth of breast cancer cells and may also offer protection against the spread of cancer, an attribute that may make it a good cancer therapy option when combined with other drugs. Just 2 $^1/_2$ cups of broccoli a week is all you need to reduce your risk of several cancers, particularly those of the breast and prostate. Broccoli also offers a healthy hit of fiber, minerals and vitamins.

Fabulous Flaxseed

Flaxseed is full of lignans—phytoestrogenic compounds that have been proven to help protect us against certain kinds of cancers, especially breast, prostate and colon. Adding 2 to 3 tablespoons of flaxseed to your smoothies, oatmeal, salads or cereals daily can reduce your cancer risk and also provide a dose of fiber and essential fatty acids. The oils in flaxseed can go rancid quickly, so be sure to purchase ground flaxseed in a vacuum-sealed package and store it in the freezer. Better yet, you can grind your own daily.

Glorious Green Tea: 4 Cups a Day

Drink 4 cups of this tasty tea daily, and you can enjoy weight loss, possibly even without a change in diet and exercise. A 1999 study published in the *American Journal of Clinical Nutrition* reported that green tea extract can significantly increase metabolism and fat burning. Questioning whether some of these effects were due to the caffeine content of green tea, the researchers delved deeper and discovered that other properties besides caffeine were behind the fat-burning benefits. While the caffeine does provide an energizing boost, the tea also offers calming effects because it contains theanine, a natural compound that blocks the release of cortisol—great for conquering ab fat!

Green tea also contains a group of antioxidants called polyphenols, which are useful for cancer protection, free radical protection and cutting inflammation, so drink plenty of it regularly. It can even help lower cholesterol and improve your blood sugar balance too.

Revel in Red Wine

The French have had it right for centuries. Consumed in moderation, red wine can reduce the risk of type 2 diabetes, prostate cancer and heart disease. The antioxidant polyphenols found in the skins and seeds of grapes, especially catechins and resveratrol, aid heart health, inhibit inflammation and help prevent the development of certain cancers. Resveratrol, a natural antifungal and antibacterial compound within grapes, may also benefit nerve cells and assist in the prevention of Alzheimer's disease and Parkinson's disease.

According to researchers from Northwestern University Medical School, many benefits of resveratrol are in fact due to its estrogenic properties. When consumed with or after a meal, red wine is a good digestive aid. Despite all the wonderful benefits of red wine, note that you should stay away from it if you have a medical condition worsened by alcohol, such as alcoholism, elevated triglycerides, pancreatitis, liver disease, uncontrolled hypertension, depression or congestive heart failure. Furthermore, even healthy individuals should limit wine intake to 2 to 3 glasses a week.

WHICH RED WINE SHOULD YOU CHOOSE?
Researchers at the University of California, Davis, tested a variety of wines to determine which types have the highest concentrations of flavonoids. They found drier wines such as cabernet sauvignon to be the flavonoid favorites, followed closely by petit syrah and pinot noir. Merlots and red zinfandels were found to have fewer flavonoids than the others.

Get Your Daily Dose of Extra-Virgin Olive Oil

Olive oil has been a vital component in a heart-healthy, Mediterranean-style diet for a millennia. The fresh news is the many additional benefits of olive oil that support its designation as a Hot Hormone food.

Olives and olive oil are rich in antioxidant compounds called polyphenols, which are known to have anti-inflammatory, anticancer and anticoagulant benefits. Olive oil also provides a rich source of plant sterols to curb inflammation, aid hormonal balance and control cholesterol. But the various ways olive oil benefits weight loss are most exciting. And these effects are not only because of its ability to reduce inflammation.

When we include them in our daily diet, monounsaturated fats such as olive oil encourage the release of our appetite-suppressing hormone leptin. Olive oil, in particular, has been shown to improve our sensitivity to insulin. In a study published in *Diabetes Care* (July 2007), 11 subjects with insulin resistance and increased abdominal fat used three different diets for 28 days. Each diet had equal calories but different compositions: one was a high-saturated-fat diet, the second was high in carbohydrates and the third was rich in monounsaturated fats. At the end of the 28-day period, researchers measured the effects of each diet on body-fat distribution, insulin resistance and adiponectin levels. (Adiponectin is a hormone released by our fat cells and known to improve insulin sensitivity, reduce inflammation and protect against obesity and metabolic syndrome.)

Can you guess the results? Of the three diets, the one rich in olive oil showed the best outcome, preventing not only belly fat accumulation but also insulin resistance and a drop in adiponectin typically seen in people who eat a high-carbohydrate diet.

Besides helping us lose weight, balance our hormones, reduce inflammation and keep insulin under control, olive oil also breaks down fat cells we already have. In a study published in the *British Journal of Nutrition* (December 2003), researchers fed three different diets to rats—one rich in olive oil, another high in polyunsaturated soybean oil and a third high in saturated fat from palm kernel oil. The results showed increased breakdown of fats within fat cells with the olive oil–rich diet. Interestingly, the *opposite* effect was noted with the diet high in soybean oil, which is one of the hormone-hindering foods we should avoid 100 percent of the time. Based on these results, staying away from soybean oil is *definitely* a good thing.

Enjoy Avocado

Avocados contain glutathione, one of the most potent antioxidants and disease-fighting agents. These rich-tasting fruits are also high in heart-friendly vitamin E and potassium. Back in 1996, avocados gained publicity as a healthy food when a study looking at the health benefits of daily avocado consumption was published in the *Archives of Medical Research*. During the study, 45 people ate avocados every day for a week (however, I recommend only $^1/_4$ of an avocado as a serving). They experienced an average 17 percent drop in total blood cholesterol and their cholesterol ratio also changed in a healthy way: LDL went down and HDL went up. Researchers now know that avocados are rich in beta-sitosterol, a natural substance shown to significantly lower blood cholesterol levels. In an article published in the *American Journal of Medicine* (December 1999), researchers pointed out that beta-sitosterol was shown to reduce cholesterol in 16 human studies. Another wonderful benefit of beta-sitosterol is that it helps to balance cortisol, even during exercise. It may also help to restore low DHEA and decrease the inflammation typically associated with the stress of intense exercise.

Unfortunately avocados earned an undeserved bad rap during the low-fat craze because they are high in monounsaturated fats. But remember, you *need* fats—healthy fats—for fat loss. Besides offering an excellent source of healthy fat, avocados are also rich in antioxidants that are great for your complexion.

An Organic Apple a Day

With all its fiber and antioxidant power, an apple a day truly can help keep the doctor away. Apples contain quercetin, a flavonoid antioxidant and natural antihistamine. Like many other flavonoids, quercetin also has phytoestrogenic properties. Finnish researchers finally completed a study in September 2002 in which 10,054 people ate an apple a day beginning in 1966! Published in the *American Journal of Clinical Nutrition*, the results showed that this simple dietary habit reduced the risk of almost every chronic disease associated with aging, including osteoporosis, heart disease, cancer, stroke, type 2 diabetes and asthma. Numerous other studies support the cancer-protective benefits of quercetin for the prostate, lung, breast and skin. For all these reasons and more, an apple a day is part of the *Supercharged Hormone Diet* nutrition plan. It must be organic because apples are one of the foods most heavily sprayed with pesticides.

Cheers for Chia Seed

Chia seed is a gluten-free ancient grain that can be added to just about any food. On a per gram basis, chia seed is touted to be:

- The highest source of omega-3s in nature with 65 percent of its total fat from omega-3 fatty acids.
- The highest source of fiber in nature—35 percent (90 percent of which is insoluble and 10 percent of which is soluble).
- Abundant in the minerals magnesium, potassium, folic acid, iron and calcium.
- A complete source of all essential amino acids and bioavailable protein.
- A great choice for a carbohydrate-conscious eater. The carbs found in chia seeds are mostly insoluble fiber, which means they have few calories and are terrific for digestion.

Just 3 1/2 ounces of chia seed offers an amazing 20 g of omega-3s, the equivalent of 1 3/4 pounds of Atlantic salmon. Wow! And then there are the hormonal benefits: chia seed stabilizes blood sugar, manages the effects of diabetes, improves insulin sensitivity and aids symptoms related to metabolic syndrome, including imbalances in cholesterol, blood pressure and high blood sugar after meals. Chia seed is highly anti-inflammatory and reduces high-sensitivity C-reactive protein, a blood marker of inflammation. This wondrous little grain also contains high amounts of tryptophan, the amino acid precursor of serotonin and melatonin.

Sure sounds like we should all be enjoying chia seed every day. It also has very little taste, which makes it easy to blend with other foods.

Go Nuts

Raw nuts such as almonds and walnuts are an excellent choice for healthy, filling snacks. Nuts are not only rich in healthy oils, zinc, selenium and vitamin E, but provide a mix of protein and carbohydrate all in one, making them a good option for the carbohydrate-conscious eater looking to lose weight. (But remember, just a small handful will do.) The healthy fats in nuts also stimulate leptin release, which helps control your appetite. Snacking on nuts or adding them to salads or oatmeal five times a week is proven to reduce your risk of type 2 diabetes and to lower cholesterol too.

Like avocados, most nuts are an excellent source of the plant sterol beta-sitosterol. Almonds, in particular, contain protein, fiber, plant sterols and several other heart-healthy nutrients. Almonds are also known to slow the absorption of carbohydrates in the body, which may help with diabetes management. In addition to lowering cholesterol levels and reducing the risk of coronary heart disease, researchers at the University of Toronto found that eating almonds may reduce the impact of carbohydrate-rich foods on blood sugar. Their data highlight that eating almonds together with carbs slows the rise in blood sugar, which may increase satiety and help keep insulin levels from fluctuating.

Here's a surprising fact about walnuts. Research from the University of Texas Health Science Center published in *Nutrition* (September 2005) showed that walnuts are a source of melatonin. You will recall that melatonin improves our sleep and offers antioxidant protection. So walnuts just might be your secret weapon against sleepless nights, as well as cancer, Parkinson's disease, Alzheimer's disease and cardiovascular illness.

And let's not forget about pecans, the only nut cited by the US Department of Agriculture in its list of "Top 20 Fruits, Vegetables and Nuts" for sources of food antioxidants. Loma Linda University also published research results in 2006 showing that adding just a handful of pecans to a balanced diet could help manage our bad LDL cholesterol. Good news for nut lovers, because pecans sure are tasty.

Soy: An Organic Non-GMO Serving Once a Day

Bone density, hormonal balance and cholesterol levels change as we age, but a daily serving of soy can help lower cholesterol, keep bones strong, improve heart health, protect the prostate and ease the symptoms of menopause. The therapeutic effects of soy products, when consumed in moderation, come from the phytoestrogens naturally present in soybeans. Just 1 cup of unsweetened, organic soy milk or yogurt, a handful of soy nuts or a palm-size serving of tempeh can do the trick. Research from the University of Illinois also suggests soy protein may help to increase metabolism, manage weight and limit the growth of fat cells. Don't go for soy, however, if you've noticed it has caused gas, bloating or digestive problems in the past.

Refreshing Reverse-Osmosis Water

Our skin certainly needs healthy fats to stay supple, but water is the key to preventing fine lines and a dehydrated appearance. Our skin, like most tissues in our body, is mostly water. Sufficient water is crucial for preventing joint stiffness, weight gain, headaches, decreased athletic performance and poor recovery after exercise. In general, the 8 cups-a-day guideline is sufficient, but you should definitely drink more when you exercise or spend time in the sun. Dehydration also increases the release of hormones, which stimulates our appetite. So next time you feel hungry, drink a glass of water first to be sure your body isn't tricking you into consuming extra calories. If you purchase water, look for reverse-osmosis or pure spring water in glass bottles rather than plastic. Also, be aware that distilled water is void of essential minerals.

Powerful Whey Protein Isolate

This powdered supplement is the most bioavailable source of protein we can get, making it a great addition to smoothies and shakes. Your liver loves whey protein because it offers a concentrated source of glutathione, just like lovely avocados. Whey has been proven to promote fat loss, preserve muscle tissue, enhance immunity, aid insulin sensitivity and support recovery after exercise. It is also a source of tryptophan, which can help raise serotonin and combat stress. For all these reasons, and more, it is an essential component of the Hormone Diet plan.

Bountiful Berries

Berries have gained plenty of good publicity as a super food choice for protection against free radicals and inflammation, both of which accelerate aging and contribute to diseases such as cancer and Alzheimer's. Blueberries, in particular, can protect us against sun damage and support eye health. They are high in fiber, low in sugar and contain a potent dose of proanthocyanidins, which are beneficial for skin, cognitive function and cardiovascular health. Blueberries may also help lower blood sugar levels and insulin resistance, as researchers in Canada have found. In a small study, overweight men at risk of heart disease and diabetes drank 1 cup of wild blueberry juice every day for 3 weeks. Their blood sugar dropped by roughly 10 percent, and their insulin resistance also fell compared with that of control-group participants who drank a placebo. The benefits may come from the effect of the fruits' high levels of anthocyanins on the pancreas, which regulates blood sugar by producing insulin.

FOOD FOR YOUR THOUGHTS
Blueberries, tea, grapes and cocoa enhance memory in mice, according to research published in *The Journal of Neuroscience* (May 2007). The effects of these foods were intensified when the mice also exercised regularly. The compound common to all these foods is epicatechin, a flavonoid that has already been shown to improve cardiovascular function and increase blood flow in the brain. Epicatechin promotes structural and functional changes in the dentate gyrus, a part of the brain involved in the formation of learning and memory. Flavonoids are also found in some chocolate, so maybe we should snack on a square before our workouts for an extra brain boost!

Most of us are familiar with blueberries and other berries typically found in our local supermarket. But have you ever heard of the açaí berry (pronounced ah-sy-ee)? Researchers at the University of Florida have recently shown these tropical berries to be even higher in antioxidants than blueberries. How about goji berries? They're also one of my new favorite snacks. Very high in fiber and antioxidants, they also contain an amazing 4 g of protein per serving and a bit of iron too! A tablespoon or two of goji berries mixed with low-fat, organic cottage cheese is a fantastic snack.

Sprinkle on the Cinnamon

I encourage you to add cinnamon to your food and hot drinks as often as possible, not only because it tastes so nice but also because it offers wonderful insulin-balancing effects. A study published in the journal *Diabetes Care* (December 2003) showed that cinnamon may cause muscle and liver cells to respond more readily to insulin. Better response to insulin means better blood sugar balance and, therefore, less insulin in your body. Cinnamon also seems to reduce several risk factors for cardiovascular disease, including high blood sugar, triglycerides, LDL cholesterol and total cholesterol. Just $1/2$ teaspoon a day for 30 days is enough to significantly improve your insulin response *and* trim your waistline. I add it to my coffee, and you should too.

Beneficial Oat Bran

Oats are a good source of many nutrients including vitamin E, zinc, selenium, copper, iron, manganese and magnesium. They are also packed with protein and fiber, which can help balance blood sugar and insulin while reducing cholesterol and heart disease risk. According to the American Cancer Society, the phytochemicals in oats may also have cancer-fighting properties. They make a nice, comfy hot snack and can easily be added to many recipes.

The Beauty of Buckwheat

Buckwheat offers us an alternative to wheat, one of the most highly allergenic foods and the grain we tend to most commonly overeat.

Buckwheat is a gluten-free grain, making it an excellent choice for those with celiac disease, gluten sensitivities, food allergies or anyone undertaking an anti-inflammatory detox. It can be used as an alternative to rice or served as porridge.

Buckwheat is higher in protein and fiber than other grains. Recall the benefits of protein: it assists with healthy immunity, healing after exercise, maintaining stable blood sugar balance and encouraging fat loss. Buckwheat is also lower on the glycemic index and results in less insulin release after consumption compared with other starches such as rice, wheat and corn, which are higher on the glycemic scale. Buckwheat is known to lower cholesterol and is a rich source of magnesium. Rich in anti-inflammatory flavonoids (especially rutin, which tones veins and is useful for treating and preventing spider or varicose veins), buckwheat is a beautiful choice for bolstering the health of our heart and blood vessels. You can find buckwheat flour or pastas at your local grocery or health-food store.

Say Yes to Plain Organic Yogurt

As a natural source of probiotics, yogurt promotes good digestion, restores healthy bacterial balance in the gut, aids the metabolism of estrogen and supports healthy immunity. Studies have shown that just $^1/_2$ cup a day can lessen the frequency and severity of colds and flus.

Besides reducing the uncomfortable abdominal bloating often associated with unsettled digestion, yogurt may also help trim your waistline by encouraging weight loss. Recent reports showing the benefits of high-calcium, low-fat dairy products for weight loss is certainly welcome news for dieters. Yogurt is a great example of a helpful food that sends the strong message to your brain that you're full. Opt for an unsweetened version. If you are lactose intolerant or have other sensitivities to dairy, however, you should leave this one out of your diet.

Pour on the Pomegranate

Researchers at the University of Wisconsin have shown that pomegranate extract has anticancer, anti-inflammatory and antioxidant properties that are effective in suppressing cancer of the skin, breast and colon. New research indicates that pomegranate may be particularly helpful for the prevention of breast cancer. The most powerful estrogen in the body, estradiol, plays an important role in the origin and development of breast cancers, most of which are hormone dependent in their early stages. Pomegranates possess natural compounds that inhibit the enzyme in women's bodies that converts the weak estrogen, estrone, into its most potent metabolite, estradiol. High amounts of this enzyme can be an indicator of adverse prognosis in women with estrogen-receptor-positive breast tumors. As a result, pomegranate offers some hope for possible therapeutic interventions in breast cancer. Guys, it's also showing promise for prostate cancer protection too. Pure pomegranate juices or seeds are a great way to enjoy the healthy benefits of this tasty ruby-red fruit.

Spice up Your Life

Herbs and spices certainly add zesty flavor to our meals, but many also offer anti-inflammatory, antioxidant, antiaging, immune-enhancing and hormone-balancing effects. Garlic, rosemary, thyme, turmeric, ginger, cumin, curry and cayenne pepper are particularly beneficial. Below are my two favorites of the bunch:

Turmeric (also called curcumin) is one of my personal favorites because it naturally reduces inflammation, pain and swelling. According to trials conducted at Johns Hopkins University School of Medicine in 2006, a combination of turmeric and quercetin, a powerful antioxidant found in onions, apples and cabbage, can help shrink painful colon polyps. Those who participated in this study experienced a 60 percent drop in the number of polyps along with 50 percent shrinkage of polyps that remained. In a 2006 study published in the *Journal of Alzheimer's Disease,* researchers at UCLA also found that turmeric helps clear the brain of the plaques that are characteristic of the disease. Incredible!

Ginger is another fabulous herb proven to prevent and treat nausea from motion sickness, pregnancy and chemotherapy. It's a potent antioxidant that works by blocking the potentially nauseating effects of serotonin on the gut. Like turmeric, ginger possesses natural anti-inflammatory benefits and may improve blood flow. A study conducted at the University of Miami showed ginger extract also had a significant effect on reducing the pain of osteoarthritis. Similarly encouraging results were found in a 2006 study at the University of Michigan Comprehensive Cancer Center. These researchers found powdered ginger killed ovarian cancer cells just as well or *better* than traditional chemotherapy.

Delicious Dark Chocolate: A 1" Square Daily

A research team from the University of Helsinki, Finland, asked pregnant women to rate their stress levels and document their chocolate consumption. Guess what they found? Six months after birth, the mothers rated their infants' behavior in various categories including fear, soothability, smiling and laughter. The babies born to women who had eaten chocolate daily during pregnancy smiled and laughed more and were more active. Even the babies of stressed women who had regularly consumed chocolate during pregnancy showed less fear of new situations than babies of stressed moms-to-be who abstained. Awesome news for new moms *and* chocoholics!

Who says we can't indulge a little and improve our health at the same time? This tasty treat boosts our endorphins and also contains tryptophan (a building block of serotonin) and the brain chemical phenylethylamine, known to promote our feelings of attraction, excitement and love. But new research shows yet another chemical is involved in the happy little high we get from chocolate. Dr. Daniele

Piomelli, a neuroscientist and professor of pharmacology at the University of California, Irvine, suggests that chocolate influences anandamide, a chemical that targets our brain much the way the active ingredient THC in marijuana does. Chocolate contains anandamide, as well as two chemicals known to slow the breakdown of this neurochemical. So it might work by prolonging the action of this natural stimulant in our brain.

Chocolate is also good for our heart and blood vessels. According to a study published in the *Journal of the American Medical Association* (July 2007), eating a small portion of dark chocolate each day can lower blood pressure without packing on extra pounds. Dark chocolate's heart-healthy effects are thought to come from flavonoids, natural compounds in cocoa beans that give dark chocolate its bittersweet taste. Dark chocolate is richest in flavonoids, whereas white chocolate contains none. Flavonoids have been shown to inhibit blood clot formation, ease constriction of blood vessels and slow the oxidation of LDL cholesterol.

Indulge in All the Hot Hormone Foods

How's this for short and sweet? Eat and enjoy as many Hot Hormone foods as you can, as often as you can! Except the chocolate, of course.

HORMONE DIET SUCCESS STORY: MITCH

"I was your typical healthy 40-something—or so I thought, until I had my blood work done! Like many of us, my poor diet, lack of exercise and stress levels had caused my cholesterol, blood pressure and sugars to creep in the wrong direction. My doctor started naming a multitude of prescription drugs to lower my blood pressure and cholesterol levels. I was not only scared—I felt old.

"The very next week I started the Hormone Diet. I found Dr. Turner to be bright, motivating and very knowledgeable. She became a partner and supporter, and she made it clear that I could fix my issues if I committed to diet, exercise, stress management and supplements. Within 4 months I saw incredible results in how I felt, how I looked, and more importantly, my stats and blood values.

MITCH

STATS	SEPT.	DEC.	LOST
Weight (in.)	173	162	11
Waist (in.)	37.8	33	4.8
Hip (in.)	41	38	3
Cholesterol (mg/dL)	295	169	125
BP	160/100	120/84	↓
Body Fat	20%	15%	5%

"It is now 9 months later, I am 20 pounds lighter, in my best shape and my blood work is picture perfect. Dr. Turner's program takes commitment, but if I can do it with three young kids and a very active business life, anyone can. The way we eat and live makes us sick, while following a healthier lifestyle can make huge changes to the way you live and feel!"

CHAPTER 8

DON'T GO TO THE
GROCERY STORE WITHOUT ME

*Build upon strengths, and weaknesses will
gradually take care of themselves.*

JOYCE C. LOCK

Now that you are armed with plenty of knowledge about which foods
to stock up on and which ones to avoid, you are ready to head to the
grocery store!

Once you have learned the basics of shopping for hormonal
health, you just might start to think of it as a challenging and fun
activity too. I love the excitement of finding a new healthy choice that
is high in fiber, low in carbs, high in protein or low in fat.

Unfortunately, my husband doesn't share in my enthusiasm. He
can't stand food shopping with me because he says I spend too much
time reading labels. Although my time spent perusing the food aisles
may seem like an inconvenience for him, it's definitely beneficial for
you. Now your grocery shopping time can be streamlined, since I have
outlined in this chapter your best choices in each section in the grocery store. I've even distinguished between brands, sometimes even
flavors within the same brand, and I've noted how each product is
categorized as one of your best options for hormonal health. I expect
we will keep building this list, so please do share your good grocery
finds with me often through drnatashaturner.com.

Shopping for Your Hormonally Balanced Diet

Before we move on to the shopping list, I would like to help you
understand the criteria behind products that receive the Hormone

Diet seal of approval. All of the products listed in this chapter possess one or more of these attributes:

- All are free of harmful fats, vegetable oil, hydrogenated oils, soybean oil, cottonseed oil and peanut oil; most contain minimal to no safflower or sunflower oil.
- Most, if not all, of the products have no sugar added.
- All are free of artificial sweeteners and harmful sugar substitutes. Only products sweetened with stevia or sugar alcohols (xylitol, erythritol) are recommended.
- I have checked the protein and carbohydrate ratio of all of the products. This list includes the products I found that were the lowest in carbs and highest in protein.
- After checking the protein and carbohydrate content, I then selected products for you that are lowest in fat and highest in fiber.

Even though I have done the label reading and product selection work for you, I believe that it is important for you to understand how to read nutrition labels. This was an enlightening experience even for me. I truly could not believe the variation in the amount of protein, carbs and fats in similar products. For example, in the veggie burger section, one product contained over 50 g of carbohydrate per burger, while another brand had less than 10! Wow! Wouldn't you want to know which brand to select that could help you lose weight and improve hormonal balance almost effortlessly? I sure would!

Understanding nutrition labels and the glycemic index will help you be carb-conscious when you shop, cook and eat. Just follow these guidelines regarding nutrition labels.

1. **Read the ingredients.** If the product contains any hormone-hindering ingredients you must avoid 100 percent of the time (see page 91), put it back on the shelf.
2. **Next move on to the nutrition label information and first check the serving size allocated for the nutrition info.** A serving size

of five potato chips doesn't make much sense based on the amount that most of us would really eat in a sitting. Sometimes foods look as though they are a good choice, but only because the serving size used to report the nutrition values is completely unrealistic.

3. **Check the amount of carbohydrate.** Read the amount listed on the label and measure it against the total amount of carbohydrate you should consume per meal and snack, noted below (these are the only numbers you *must* memorize, I promise!). If the product is higher than these amounts, look for something else. I also want you to compare the amount of carbohydrate relative to protein (see below).

4. **Check the amount of protein.** Remember this simple guideline: if the product contains similar amounts of protein and carbohydrate or, even better, more protein than carbs per serving, it is a good choice for you. For example: vanilla soy milk has 11 g of carbs and 6 g of protein; plain soy milk has 3 g of carbs and 6 g of protein. In this case, the plain milk is a much better bet.

5. **Next check the fat content.** Compare it with the total amount of fat you should consume in a meal or snack (again, noted below). Check the saturated fat content, in particular, and aim for little to none, but certainly no more than 3 g per serving. Here's another guideline for hormonal health: high protein supersedes low fat. So if you have to decide between a product that has more protein but also slightly more fat over another that has lower protein as well as low fat, I suggest that you still go for the higher protein option for the most metabolic benefits.

6. **Check the fiber content.** Products that contain less than 2 g of fiber per serving are not great choices. If you have a number of brands to choose from, select the product that's highest in fiber (and, if possible, also lowest in carbs and highest in protein).

7. **Check the sodium content.** Products with less than 140 mg of salt per serving are considered to be low-sodium choices. Remember, you should consume only 2,300 mg of sodium per day, which is equal to about a teaspoon of table salt. When comparing products, pick the one that's lowest in sodium. Sometimes I may end up consuming more sodium if the product happens to have a great protein and carb balance. Just remember to keep up your water intake, and avoid high-sodium options completely if you have high blood pressure.

8. **Check the calorie content.** Measure the calorie count against the total number of calories you should be having. About 500 calories per meal is a good guideline.

Becoming familiar with your best low-glycemic carbohydrates, as outlined in the chart showing your allowed foods for week 4 in Part Two, together with learning to read labels effectively, will arm you with all the information you need to be truly nutritionally savvy. You will be able to make great choices no matter where you are or what you are up to.

Here are the only numbers you need to memorize for this whole book! You should stick to the serving sizes listed in your chart in Part Two for the foods to enjoy for the Glyci-Med approach, or use these guidelines when eating something that has a nutrition label:

WOMEN		MEN	
MEALS (3)	SNACKS (2)	MEALS (3)	SNACKS (2–3)
Protein: 25–30 g	10–20 g	Protein: 35–40 g	15–25 g
Carbs: 20–30 g	10–15 g	Carbs: 35–40 g	15–20 g
Fats: 10–14 g	6–7 g	Fats: 13–17 g	7–8 g

You may choose to have four regular-size meals or three meals and two snacks.

Ultimately these numbers translate to a diet comprising the following macronutrient ratios:

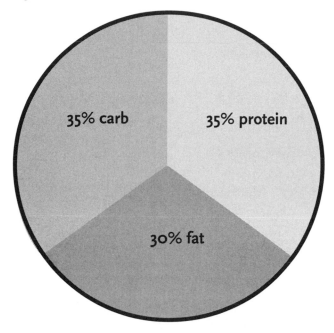

A Few of My Favorite Brands

Both my professional practice and my personal commitment to healthy eating have led me to discover some excellent products that are available in health-food stores and, I am pleased to report, in more and more mainstream supermarkets. You certainly do not need to purchase all of the items listed in each section below. My goal is to help make your shopping easier by recommending some of my favorites that you could try next time you venture down the grocery aisle.

Keep in mind that product ingredients (as well as calorie and carb counts) might differ slightly depending on the country that you are shopping in. Be sure to check your labels and be sure to avoid those with the following: soy oil, cottonseed oil, vegetable oil and partially hydrogenated oil. Happy shopping!

Wholesome Sweeteners

One of the rules of the Hormone Diet is to avoid added sugar. But I also emphasize that you stay away from artificial sweeteners, which can increase your appetite, cravings, blood sugar and insulin. Instead, look for these natural alternatives when you need a little boost of sweetness:

Coconut Secret—raw coconut crystals
> Low-GI, low-calorie sweetener
> 1 tablespoon = 7 g sugar/carbs

Wholesome Sweeteners Zero
> Made with organic erythritol, this sweetener contains zero carbs and is diabetic friendly.

Yacon Pro—Organic Yacon Syrup
> Not sugar-free, but contains only 7.35 g of carbs per serving.

Eden Organic Apple Butter
> Another option for a sweetener, but it is not calorie- or carb-free.
> 1 tablespoon = 20 calories
> 4 g sugar

Xylitol USA (Xyla)
> If you haven't heard of this company you will soon. With everything from ketchup and barbeque sauce to jam and chocolate, their products are safe for diabetes, gluten-free, low sodium and free of artificial sweeteners. Instead, they use Xylitol, which has a low-glycemic impact, fewer calories, is great for your teeth and waist-friendly. Their ketchup will have you forgetting about the good old-fashioned one—and it pours faster out of the bottle. One tablespoon is 10 calories, with 3 g of carbs (2 g of that from sugar alcohols). Their Xyla mints are another tasty great option.

Cereals

I am not really a fan of cereals, especially for breakfast, but there are some selections that are more Hormone Diet friendly than others. Here are your best choices:

Food for Life Ezekiel 4:9

Much like their flourless yeast-free sprouted grain breads, these cereals are rich in protein, vitamins, minerals and natural fiber with no added fat. A $1/2$ cup serving is 200 calories, 3 g of fat, 8 g of protein and 38 g of carbs (6 g of that in fiber). I recommend using a $1/3$ cup and topping it with additional protein such as Greek yogurt and fats such as 1 teaspoon of almond slivers.

Trader Joe's Steel Cut Organic Oats

If the detox process gave you the green light to include oats in your diet, then my favorite would have to be the steel cut variety. It comes in a regular and a "quick cook" version, and $1/4$ cup measured dry amount has 150 calories, 2.5 g of fat, 5 g of protein and 27 g of carbs (including 4 g of fiber).

McCann's Steel Cut Oats

This is the lowest carbohydrate oatmeal I have found. It has 25 g of carbs, 5 g of protein, and 4 g of fiber per serving. Half a serving is good for a snack. Don't forget to add your protein.

Nature's Path Foods—Kamut Puffs

A 1-cup serving of this cereal contains only 11 g of carbs along with 2 g of fiber and 2 g of protein. Perhaps one of the nicest attributes of this product is that it contains 100 percent kamut and nothing else!

Nature's Path Foods—Millet Rice Flakes

Wheat-free and contains 22 g of carbs, 3 g of fiber and 4 g of protein per serving.

Barbara's Bakery Multigrain Shredded Spoonfuls

Lower in carbs than most other cereals, this option contains 23 g of carbs along with 1.5 g of fat, 3 g of fiber and 3 g of protein per serving.

Nature's Path Foods—Smart Bran with Psyllium

A $2/3$-cup serving of this cereal contains 24 g of carbs, which is higher than desired, but it also has a whopping 8 g of fiber! Protein and fat are on the low side at 3 g and 1.5 g, respectively.

Kellogg's All-Bran Original (¹/₂ cup)

Definitely the star when it comes to being a source of fiber, with a whopping 12 g per serving! It does contain 27 g of carbs and only 4 g of protein, but it is low in fat at only 1 g.

Nature's Path—FlaxPlus Multibran (³/₄ cup)

A decent source of fiber (5 g) and low in fat (1.5 g), but it's slightly high in carbs (23 g) and low in protein (4 g).

Nutritious Living Hi-Lo

This cereal is tops for its protein and carb content. It contains only 13 g of carbs per serving and a fabulous 12 g of protein. It's also high in fiber (6 g) and low in fat (1 g).

Nutritious Living Hi-Lo with Strawberries is very similar but has just 1 extra gram of carbs for a total of 14 g per serving.

Breads, Pastas and Flours

Finn Crisp

Their organic sourdough rye crispbread is baked with organically farmed rye and contains no additives. One slice is just 90 calories, 3.8 g of carbs (1.3 g of that is fiber) and 0.2 g of fat. Suitable for vegetarians, their products contain no lactose, soy milk or eggs. Their non-organic varieties include wheat in the ingredients (so watch for allergies) and come in multigrain, caraway-kummin, coriander and garlic flavors.

Kavli Crispy Thin Crispbread

If you are a fan of crispbread, of course, your detox process gave the green light for rye products, you can't go wrong with this Norwegian whole grain option. Famous for its naturally crisp texture and mild nutty taste, 3 pieces (15 g) are just 50 calories, 0 g of fat and 11 g of carbs. Add a high-protein cheese and a handful of nuts for a snack.

Food for Life—Ezekiel 4:9

If you are craving raisin toast, the Cinnamon Raisin variety is your best bet. It's a lovely treat when toasted and topped with almond butter. Your best selection from a carb perspective is the Ezekiel Sesame. It contains only 14 g of carbs and offers 3 g of fiber.

You can also select the Ezekiel tortillas, cereal, hot dog buns and burger buns.

Sobaya Kamut and Buckwheat Pasta (3 ounces)

Although still high in carbohydrates (59 g per serving), the Kamut and Buckwheat Pasta is much higher in fiber (4 g) and protein (11 g) than other types of pasta. It is also wheat-free.

The Kamut Pasta has a similar nutrition profile at 5 g of fiber, 10 g of protein and 57 g of carbs.

King Soba—Organic Brown Rice and Wakame Noodles (1.9 ounces)

A wheat- and gluten-free option. This product contains 36 g of carbs, 3 g of fiber and 6 g of protein per serving. Keep your serving size small, otherwise you will consume too many carbohydrates. The 100 percent buckwheat type has 8 g of protein, 5 g of fiber and is slightly lower in carbs at 33 g.

Eden Organic Pasta Company—Kamut Spirals (3 ounces)

With 8 g of fiber, 51 g of carbs and 14 g of protein, this pasta is an OK choice. It's also 100 percent whole grain with no added salt, and it is certified kosher. Much like the soba noodles, you will want to keep your portions low to avoid taking in too many carbs.

Maranatha

This brand is fairly easy to find in a grocery store and usually a staple in any health food store. With a range of options from raw to regular almond butter, Maranatha achieves with a creamy versus soupy consistency. One tablespoon is 95 calories, 8 g of fat and 7 g of carbs (with 3 g of those being fibrous). As with all nut butters, avoid those with added sugars.

Artisana

The quickest way to alter the flavor of your morning smoothie and avoid breakfast boredom is to frequently change the fat source, and that includes nut butters. Artisana is made in a vegan facility and offers organic raw nut butters, from almond to cashews. One tablespoon completes your fat requirement for a meal or smoothie with 90 calories, 8 g of fat, 8 g of carbs and 6 g of protein for their cashew flavor.

Condiments

Pure Kraft—Greek Feta

This dressing is made with canola and olive oils and contains no sugar, so it's great both during detox and while you are on maintenance. Kraft's Creamy Balsamic flavor has only 2 g of carbs and tastes great.

Hellmann's Mayonnaise

I like Hellmann's half-fat mayonnaise, which slashes both the fat and the calories by 50 percent. It's also low in saturated fat and cholesterol and contains no trans fats. Hellmann's also makes a Bertolli Olive Oil Mayonnaise, which has a mix of mono- and polyunsaturated fats and is made from canola oil and extra-virgin olive oil.

Pickles

Pickles are a great way to spice up anything from a salad to a snack without adding a lot of carbs or calories. The key is to steer clear of the high-sodium and added sugars ones. Mt. Olive pickles have Reduced Sodium Kosher Baby Dills (135 mg per serving) and Reduced Sodium Kosher Dill Strips (120 mg per serving) with just 1 g of carbs. Real Pickles Organic Dill Pickles are available in the Northeast states and include 100 percent organic ingredients with no sugars or unpronounceable additives.

Nuts to You Nut Butter

This is one of my favorite nut butter brands. You can taste the difference, and it is not a soupy paste. Two tablespoons of almond or cashew butter contains 18 g of fat, 6 g of carbs and 5 g of protein. The pumpkin seed butter has a slightly lower 13 g of fat, a whopping 10 g of protein and only 4 g of carbs. Use 1 tablespoon for a great, gluten-free source of protein and healthy fat.

Spectrum Canola Oil Mayonnaise

This mayo is free of cornstarch, low in cholesterol and rich in heart-healthy monounsaturated fats (7 g per serving!). Stir it with smashed garlic and a squeeze of lemon or blend together with horseradish and lemon zest for an extra kick of low-calorie flavor.

Eden Organic Tamari Soy Sauce

This is a low-calorie, wheat-free soy sauce made from organic soybeans. Each tablespoon has only 10 calories, 2 g of carbs and 2 g of protein, but it also contains 990 mg of sodium, so be sure to increase your water intake if you like to use this sauce.

Bragg's All Purpose Seasoning

Also known as Bragg Liquid Aminos, this sauce is a certified non-GMO liquid protein concentrate, derived from soybeans, that contains essential and non-essential amino acids in naturally occurring amounts. It tastes very similar to regular soy sauce but is a little easier on sodium. There are 160 mg per $^1/_2$ teaspoon, but you only need to use a small amount since the taste is strong.

Omega Nutrition Apple Cider Vinegar

Apple cider vinegar has many benefits, from increasing circulation and energy to improving digestion and skin health. Best of all, it boasts 0 calories and 0 carbs.

Zukay Salad Dressings

Unique raw fermented salad dressings with 0 fat and no oils. These dressings are rich in enzymes and live cultures, which is great for your digestion as well as your taste buds.

Annie's Naturals—Balsamic Vinaigrette

This is an organic salad dressing that is also dairy-, gluten- and soy-free, so it's perfect while you are on the detox. Two tablespoons give you 100 calories, 10 g of fat and 3 g of carbs.

Crofter's Superfruit Spread

Made with ripe, organic fruit, these spreads come in a wide variety of flavors. They are sweetened with fair-trade sugar and contain one-third less sugar than regular jam. A 1-tablespoon serving contains 30 calories and 8 g of carbs (7 g from naturally occurring sugars).

Frontera Salsa

With gourmet flavors ranging from Chipotle and Habañero to Mango Key Lime and Spanish Olive, this isn't your ordinary salsa. Lucky for us it's also gluten-free. What I really like about this salsa is that it's simple with just a handful of ingredients (all that you can pronounce). Two tablespoons adds pizazz to your meal regardless of your expertise in the kitchen with just 10 calories, 3 g of carbs and 1 g of fiber.

Muir Glen Organic

From tomato sauce to salsa, this company provides an assortment of all-natural, organic products that taste homemade all the while focusing on organic, sustainable agriculture. Add a dash of flavor with black bean and corn, medium chipotle, media garlic cilantro or get back to the basics with good old-fashioned medium or mild salsa. Two tablespoons of salsa have 20 calories, 4 g of carbs and just 1 g of sugar.

Trader Jose's Salsa Verde

Top your proteins with this spicy, lime-flavored salsa and you can skip the preservatives and thickening agents. Made with fresh tomatillos and jalapeños, 2 tablespoons is just 10 calories, however, there are 280 mg of sodium so more isn't necessarily better in this case.

Sauces/Flavoring

The Ginger People

The Ginger Peanut Sauce is a rich, nutty and yummy complement for chicken or beef kabobs. Sweetened with cider vinegar and natural cane juice, each 2-tablespoon serving has only 25 calories, 4 g of carbs and 2 g of sugar. The Ginger Sesame Sauce is 40 calories per ounce (30 g), with 3.5 g of fat and 2.5 g of carbs. Avoid both if you have a sensitivity to soy, wheat or peanuts.

Thai Kitchen

I like their red curry and green curry pastes, as they are gluten-free with no added sugar or harmful oils. The former has 25 calories and 4 g of carbs per tablespoon, while the latter contains 10 calories and 3 g of carbs. Their organic lite coconut milk also has 60 percent fewer calories and fat than regular coconut milk.

Spreads and Dips

When it comes to spreads and dips, there are many to avoid because they have added sugar and less-than-healthy oils. For example, Simply Organic dressings and sauces use soybean oil, while Old El Paso Salsa has added sugars and hydrogenated oil.

Fontaine Santé

This company makes several dips and spreads. The veggie pâté has 4 g of protein (3 g in the traditional flavor), 3 g of carbs and 9 g of fat, so be sure to watch your serving size. The hummus comes in many flavors, and the spinach dip is made with canola oil.

Salad Dressings

Bolthouse Farms

Bolthouse Farms is one of the world's largest producers of carrots but also offers other products. Vinaigrettes come in tropical mango, classic balsamic and a raspberry merlot. Two tablespoons has only 2 g of fat and 5 g of carbs.

Private Stock by Chef Robert

These oil-based products use high-quality ingredients, have no added sugar and taste good. The company has a variety of products including:

Vinaigrettes

    Fat-Free Blueberry Pomegranate

    Mango Poppyseed

    Fat-Free Raspberry

    Asiago Caesar

    Basil Spirulina

    Mango Green Tea

    Balsamic Dijon

Crackers and Snacks

Most brand-name crackers and prepared snacks contain too much sugar and harmful fats. These selections here, however, are free of harmful oils and are much healthier options.

Mary's Organic Crackers

These organic, wheat-free and gluten-free crackers contain no harmful oils. The Original flavor is made with organic whole-grain brown rice, organic flaxseed and organic brown sesame seeds, with no added fat. Other flavors include Caraway, Black Pepper and Herb. A fulfilling 13 crackers will provide 20 g of carbs, 3 g of fiber, 3 g of protein and 3.5 g of fat.

Finn Crisp Crispbread

Choose this multi-grain cracker for its 24 g of carbs, 1.5 g of fat, 4 g of fiber and 4 g of protein per serving (5 crackers). Avoid this one, however, if you are sensitive to rye flour.

Kavli 5 Grain All Natural Whole-Grain Crispbread

These crispbreads have a mild, nutty taste. They are baked using only pure, natural ingredients; are high in fiber and low in calories; and do not contain cholesterol. Two slices gives you 14 g of carbs, 3 g of fiber and 2 g of protein. The traditional Crispy Thin is similar but has 12 g of carbs, 2 g of fiber and 1 g of protein.

Ryvita Multigrain Crispbread

These crispbreads are high in fiber, low in saturated fat and have no artificial colors or preservatives. Each slice has 6.7 g of carbs, 1.8 g of fiber, 0.6 g of fat and 1 g of protein.

Wasa Crispbread

This company makes various crispbreads that are all natural and fat-free. Each slice has approximately 10 g of carbs, 2 g of fiber and 45 calories.

Hol-Grain Crackers

These tasty crackers come in Brown Rice, Onion & Garlic, and Brown Rice & Sesame, with salt-free options. They contain no added fat, sugar, imitation flavorings, artificial ingredients or preservatives.

Dairy and Eggs

Fage Yogurt

This product line is easy to find at most grocery stores and can be used as a snack or in the preparation of dips, desserts and smoothies. I recommend their Greek yogurt, which is packed with protein, particularly their Fage Total 0% (plain) with only 100 calories, 18 g of protein and 7 carbs for a 6-ounce container. Fage Total Classic (plain) is another option that fits the bill for hormonally balanced nutrition with 190 calories, 18 g of protein and 10 g of fat per 7-ounce container.

Redwood Hills Goat Milk Yogurt

Dairy made from sheep's or goat's milk tends to cause fewer digestive issues for those who are lactose intolerance, without giving up the healthy probiotic content. One 6-ounce container from Redwood Hills has 100 calories, 4.5 g fat, 7g of carbs and 7 g of protein. Choose the plain option to steer clear of excess sugars.

Trader Joe's Goat Milk Yogurt

A popular chain with an assortment of organic options, Trader Joe's also offers a plain goat milk yogurt that's 100 calories, 4.5 g fat, 7 g carbs and 7 g of protein for a 6-ounce serving.

Trader Joe's Goat's Milk Creamy Cheese

You may be able to fool even the most dedicated cream cheese lovers with this goat's milk rendition—the main benefit is that the reduction in lactose won't aggravate your stomach. A

1-ounce serving is 45 calories, 3.5 g of fat and just 1 g of carbs. Line a couple celery stalks with this for an easy snack.

Cabot Cheese

Like my other dairy choices the key is to choose options that are particularly high in protein. Their 75% less fat Sharp Extra Light and Habañero Light cuts the fat without sacrificing flavor. It's also naturally lactose and gluten free with 60 calories, 2.5 g of fat and 9 g of protein for a 1-ounce serving. Combine 2 ounces with 1 tablespoon of nuts and an apple for a quick and easy snack.

Chobani Greek Yogurt

Greek yogurt in general livens up any smoothie and Chobani's version has less than 5 percent lactose, which makes it a feasible option for many people who usually steer clear of dairy due to digestive issues. Opt for their non-fat plain Greek yogurt with 23 g of protein for an 8-ounce serving or their low-fat plain Greek yogurt with 5 g of fat, 9 g of carbs and 22 g of protein for an 8-ounce serving. Although their flavored versions are sweetened with natural sugars such as evaporated cane juice, this will still causes spike in insulin so you should avoid them.

Organic Valley

This farmer-owned brand offers a low-fat cottage cheese made from organic milk that excludes the additives found in many competitors' products. It's also suitable for lacto-vegetarians and is certified kosher. A $^1/_2$ cup portion is just 100 calories, 2 g of fat and 4 g carbs all the while giving you 15 g of protein. Just watch for the sodium when eaten in excess (450 mg per serving).

Horizon Valley

Blending the goodness of organic dairy with live and active cultures to support digestive health, Horizon Valley offers a low fat cottage cheese with less sodium (390 mg per serving). A $^1/_2$ cup renders just 100 calories, 2.5 g of fat, 4 g of carbs and 14 g of protein. Two tablespoons of their reduced-fat cream cheese can provide another option for a fat source in your snacks with just 70 calories and 7 g of fat.

Crystal Farms All Whites

Gone are the days when you had to toss out the yolks—now it's easy to find a carton of egg whites. However, if you don't look closely, you may find a number of other ingredients sneak into the carton. All Whites is literally just that, with no additives. Three tablespoons gives you 5 g of protein and has 25 calories.

Treats—Chips, Chocolate, Frozen Desserts

Xylitol USA (Xyla)

If you haven't heard of this company you will soon. With everything from ketchup and barbeque sauce to jam and chocolate, their products are safe for diabetes, gluten-free, low sodium and free of artificial sweeteners. Instead, they use Xylitol, which has a low-glycemic impact, fewer calories, is great for your teeth and waist-friendly. Their ketchup will have you forgetting about the good old-fashioned one—and it pours faster out of the bottle. One tablespoon is 10 calories, with 3 g of carbs (2 g of that from sugar alcohols). Their Xyla mints are another tasty great option.

Trader Joe's Cocoa Powder Unsweetened

The magic of cocoa extends beyond its many health benefits. In fact, it can transform your vanilla protein shake into chocolate, add a twist to your Greek yogurt or spruce up your morning coffee. Made with tumaco cocoa powder from Columbia, 1 tablespoon is just 20 calories and 2 g of carbs (including 1 g of fiber).

Green & Black's Organic Chocolate

If you are craving something sweet, you can indulge in a small piece of this flavorful organic chocolate. All varieties are egg-free, gluten-free and suitable for vegetarians. They do contain dairy and soy, so avoid them if you have sensitivities to these ingredients.

ShaSha Co.

These certified organic cookies contain no additives and are free of trans fats and cholesterol. With flavors of Spelt Ginger Snaps and Cocoa Snaps, a serving of 15 of these little heart-shaped cookies has only 23 g of carbs, 8 g of sugar, 3 g of fat and 3 g of protein.

Cruncha Ma-Me

It's hard to turn away a high-protein, high-fiber snack that not only satisfies your urge to crunch, but also lets you reap the benefits of hormonally balanced nutrition. One 20-ounce bag of these freeze-dried edamame snacks are 90 calories, 4 g of fat, 7 g of carbs and 8 g of protein. They also come in lightly seasoned, sea salt & black pepper, onion & chive and jalapeño flavors. Enjoy two bags for a complete snack.

Organic Traditions Navitas Naturals

A tasty addition to smoothies, yogurt, fruit and even coffee, raw cocoa powder is a quick way to quench a chocolate craving and take advantage of the many antioxidant benefits. This is a healthy alternative to conventional over-processed cocoa options with 60 calories, 1.5 g fat, 9 g of carbs (4 g of that being fibrous) and 3 g of protein for every 2.5 tablespoons (14 g).

Terra Vegetable Chips

These are a lower glycemic option to the standard potato chip, because they are made from a mix of taro, sweet potato, yucca, batata, parsnip and ruby taro. They are not only colorful, but tasty as well. A 1-ounce serving has 7 g of fat and 18 g of carbs with 4 g of fiber.

Drinks and Fruit Juices

Quality fruit juices contain nutrients, but they can be very high in naturally occurring sugars. Use juices sparingly, and try mixing them with water or soda water to make a refreshing drink with fewer calories and carbs.

Recommended brands of natural fruit juices without sugar added include:

- Ceres
- Kiju
- R.W. Knudsen

- POM Wonderful
- Blue Diamond Growers

Almond Breeze

A non-dairy beverage made from real almonds. It's gluten-, cholesterol- and lactose-free and a refreshing alternative to soy and rice drinks. Choose the unsweetened, vanilla or chocolate flavors, which have only 3 g of fat, 2 g of carbs and 1 g of protein.

Zevia Natural Diet Sodas

These soft drinks are sweetened with stevia and erythritol and come in a variety of flavors, from black cherry to ginger root beer. Best of all, Zevia has no calories, no net carbohydrates and no fat. Safe for diabetics and dieters alike!

Vita Coco—Natural Coconut Water

This is a pasteurized drink made from green coconuts. Each 11-ounce serving has 15 g of carbohydrates, coming from naturally occurring sugars. Coconut water also has 15 times more potassium than that found in sport drinks (515 mg), so it's great for high-energy days.

Edensoy

Since not all soy milk is made equal, you want to be on the lookout for a brand that offers an unsweetened version made from organic non-GMO soybeans. Edensoy fits the bill with just purified water and organic soybeans in their ingredient list. A 4-ounce serving has 60 calories, 3 g fat, 2.5 g carbs and 6 g of protein—not to mention 460 mg of potassium.

Trader Joe's Coconut Water

If you haven't jumped on the coconut water bandwagon yet, it's a great water to rehydrate after a workout, add flavor to your smoothie or just quench your thirst. An 8-ounce glass is 50 calories and 12 g of carbs with a whopping 450 mg of potassium. The sugars can add up so despite it having water in the title you certainly want to limit it to 1 cup a day.

Trader Joe's Coconut Milk

The key with coconut milk is to seek out the unsweetened options. This non-dairy beverage is lactose, soy and dairy free. One cup is 50 calories, 5 g of fat, 1 g of protein and 1 g of carbs. It's also a good source of medium chain fatty acids (MCFAs), which helps to boost your metabolism.

Perrier—Lemon, Lime or Grapefruit

If you like a lemon or lime flavor, this is a great 0-calorie

---

WATCH YOUR DRINK CHOICES!

We all know we should limit sugary soft drinks. But even *so-called* healthy drinks can give us an unexpected sugar blast.

(Note: 1 teaspoon = 5 g)

*Hype per 8 ounces: 64 g

*Minute Maid Cranberry Grape per 8 ounces: 38 g

*Tropicana Twister Soda (Orange) per 8 ounces: 35 g

*Sunkist Orange Soda per 8 ounces: 35 g

*Fanta Orange per 8 ounces: 34.3 g

*Sun Drop per 8 ounces: 33 g

†Starbucks, Dulce de Leche Frappuccino Blended Crème per
    16 ounces (Grande): 85 g

†Starbucks Caffe Vanilla Frappuccino Blended Coffee
    (no whip) per 16 ounces (Grande): 67 g

‡Rockstar Energy Drink per 8 ounces: 31 g

‡Vitamin Water B-Relaxed Jackfruit and Guava Flavor per
    8 ounces: 13 g

‡Arizona Lemon Iced Tea per 8 ounces: 24 g

‡Sobe Mango Melon per 8 ounces: 29 g

‡Minute Maid Lemonade per 8 ounces: 27 g

‡Capri Sun, Pacific Cooler per 6.75 ounces: 18 g

Sources:

*energyfiend.com/sugar-in-drinks/

†starbucks.com

‡sugarstacks.com

---

beverage with only 3 mg of sodium per cup. My new favorite drink is their grapefruit flavor.

San Benedetto

Bottled right at the spring, 1,000 feet underground, San Benedetto water is rich in essential minerals with 0 calories and 0 sodium.

Tazo Teas

Commonly found and served at Starbucks, Tazo's teas have full-leaf filter bags and come in a variety of flavored green teas, black teas and herbal infusions. A great low- or caffeine-free alternative to coffee.

Stash Teas

All herbal teas can be consumed as desired.

Mighty Leaf Teas

This is another loose-leaf tea option that blends a variety of herbs and spices. Mighty Leaf's website lists the teas by flavor, mood and level of caffeine.

Almond Dream Enriched Original

This non-dairy beverage provides a source of vitamins A and E and is fortified with vitamins B12 and D and calcium. Each cup has 2.5 g of fat, 6 g of carbs and 1 g of protein. It's sweetened with organic cane juice but is also available unsweetened.

Meats, Fish and Veggie Protein

Raincoast Trading Canned Tuna

While more expensive than standard canned tuna, this company uses only eco-friendly, dolphin-safe fishing practices. The solid white albacore tuna has no salt added and 18 g of protein and 3 g of fat for each 55 g serving, making it higher in protein than most brands.

Applegate Farms Organic Turkey Burgers

This is a healthy protein source, using organic and vegetarian grain fat turkey, while packing 22 g of protein per burger. With

11 g of fat there's no need to add additional fats to your meal. Their organic turkey bacon is a great healthy alternative with 35 calories, 1.5 g of fat and 6 g of protein per slice (28 g).

Trader Joe's Organic Tofu Veggie Burgers

While tofu burgers are easy to find, the organic variety can be trickier to locate. These tasty meat substitutes use organic ingredients right down to the carrots and kale. One patty 170 calories, 12 g of fat, 7 g of carbs and 11 g of protein.

Trader Joe's Frozen Cooked Shrimp

A rule of thumb for any packaged protein: Check the labels. In this case it's nice and easy—just shrimp and salt. A serving of 3 ounces, or 7 shrimp, is just 60 calories, 1 g of fat and 14 g of protein. Simply, thaw, rinse and fry up or serve cool with a side dish for dinner.

Organic Sunshine Burgers

These delicious veggie burgers are made of sunflower seeds and contain no soy or wheat, which is ideal for gluten-free diets. Select the Original or Garden Herb flavors, with approximately 13 g of carbs, 3 g of fiber and 8 g of protein per burger. Since they are made from seeds, each burger has 13 g of fat, so avoid adding additional fats to your meal.

Lightlife Organic Tempeh

Tempeh is an excellent source of vegetarian protein that is high in fiber and low in sodium. This brand comes in Flax, Three Grain and plain soy tempeh. A 4-ounce serving is just 70 calories, 8 g of fat, 22 g of protein and 16 g of carbs, with the majority of that coming from fiber.

Amy's Kitchen Texas Burgers

This protein-rich, all-vegetarian soy burger is combined with a distinctive blend of vegetables and grains for a barbecue flavor and texture. Each patty is sweetened with cane juice and gives you 12 g of protein, 14 g of carbs, 3 g of fiber and less than 3 g of fat. Contains safflower and/or sunflower oil.

Yves Veggie Cuisine

This meatless burger comes in Bistro Chicken flavor and is a great-tasting alternative for vegetarians. It contains wheat gluten, yeast and canola oil, so avoid this product if you have sensitivities to these ingredients. Each burger provides 16 g of protein, 8 g of carbs, 3 g of fiber and less than 3 g of fat. Note that each burger has a whopping 490 mg of sodium.

Sol Cuisine Original Burger

This soy-based burger includes minimal ingredients and maximum taste. Using sunflower oil, each patty has 15 g of protein, 7 g of carbs, 4 g of fiber, 2.8 g of fat and 0 sugar. It's also lower in sodium than the Yves brand, with only 290 mg per patty.

Sol Cuisine Spicy Black Bean Burger

A delicious blend of black beans, sweet corn and Tex-Mex flavors in a soy-based burger. The burger also contains sunflower oil and is both wheat- and gluten-free. Each burger has 11 g of carbs, 4 g of fiber, 13 g of protein and 2.5 g of fat.

Whole Foods Market Burgers:

Tuna Burgers

This lightly seasoned burger is made with wild-caught yellowfin tuna with some safflower and canola oil added. Serve with homemade wasabi mayo and avocado for a tuna burger with flair. Each patty packs 21 g of protein and 0 carbs.

Alaska Salmon Burgers

Sourced from the waters off Alaska, this burger uses salmon that is MSC-certified. Serve on top of a salad or with grilled sun-dried tomatoes and basil mayo. Each patty packs 18 g of protein and 0 carbs.

Mahi Mahi Burgers

Sourced from the Pacific waters of the equator, Whole Foods mahi mahi is wild-caught and lightly seasoned for a mild but delectable flavor. Serve on lettuce with one or two grilled pine-apple slices for a truly tropical burger or mix Dijon mustard and low-sodium soy or teriyaki sauce for an Asian twist. Each patty packs 18 g of protein and 0 carbs. Mahi mahi is higher in mercury than most other fish, so enjoy only occasionally.

Protein Bars

Bars are great as meal replacements or snacks but be careful because many are loaded with added sugar, artificial sweeteners and harmful oils.

Simply Bar

These are excellent bars that are not only low glycemic, but also vegan, dairy-free, gluten-free and kosher. Available in a wide variety of flavors, they are all under 160 calories and over 16 g of protein.

Proteins+ Express Bars

A protein-rich snack with no artificial fillers or sweeteners. Choose the Natural Chocolate flavor, made with real Belgian chocolate and 14 g of protein, 24 g of carbs, 4 g of fiber and 6 g of fat.

Quest Nutrition

There are few protein bars available that can satisfy your taste-buds along with your desire for a low-glycemic, low-carb meal replacement without artificial sweeteners—Quest hits the spot. Their all natural line is sweetened with stevia versus sugar alcohols and packs 17 g of fiber, 5 to 7 g of fat and 20 g of protein. Flavors include banana nut muffin, chocolate pea-nut butter, cinnamon roll, strawberry cheesecake, lemon cream pie and, my favorite, coconut cashew.

Protein Powders

These supplements provide a very fast, easy, pure and highly absorb-able protein source. Whey protein isolate, for instance, is the most bioavailable source of protein. It supports healthy immune system function and is the most useful type of protein to encourage the loss of body fat while maintaining muscle mass. It is also a source of the antioxidant glutathione. A whey protein isolate is easier to absorb than a concentrate and tends to cause less digestive upset for individuals sensitive to dairy because it is lactose-free. Always choose protein powder supplements that are free of added sugar and artificial sweeteners. Fermented soy is also a good choice because it is easily absorbed. Jarrow makes a very good fermented soy powder that is organic, free of sweeteners and sugar, and does not contain GMO soy.

Proteins+

Containing alpha+™ whey protein isolate, proteins+ provides an absorbable source of protein with digestion enzymes, and no artificial ingredients. Two scoops contain 25 g of protein and fewer than 2 g of carbs.

Dream Protein

Amazing taste, and it mixes without a blender. A very pure product—in a 24 g scoop, 20 g of it is protein. It comes in both chocolate and vanilla flavors. The vanilla is the favorite at Clear Medicine; it's definitely one of our top-selling products.

AOR Advanced Whey

A high-quality protein with 23 g of protein, 1.4 g of carbs and 1 g of fat per scoop. This product does contain, however, a mixture of protein concentrate and isolate. So, if you are lactose intolerant, select another brand that is a 100 percent isolate.

> **THE RIGHT BLEND**
> Stock your kitchen with a blender or, even better, a Vitamix blender. You will never need to buy another blender and will be able to make the most amazing smoothies!
>
> **HOT HORMONE TIP**

Interactive Absolute Isolate Protein

Derived entirely from cross-flow micro-filtered whey protein isolate, each serving contains 25 g of protein and is exceptionally low in carbs, lactose, fat and cholesterol. It also includes an enzyme blend for enhanced digestion and is sweetened with stevia.

Nutribiotic Rice Protein

This vegetable protein is free of the common food allergens normally associated with products such as soy, milk, egg, wheat and yeast. Made from whole brown rice, each tablespoon has 0.3 g of fat, 1.8 g of carbs and 12 g of protein. Have 2 to 3 tablespoons for a full serving of protein.

Vegan Proteins+

This comprehensive formula contains a variety of vegetarian proteins including non-GMO pea, cranberry, brown rice, alfalfa and hemp. One serving provides all 8 essential amino acids, 8 vitamins, 13 minerals and 20 g of protein.

Vega Sport Natural Plant-based Protein

This product is derived from a broad spectrum blend of sprouted whole-grain brown rice, green pea, hemp, alfalfa and spirulina proteins. Each scoop contains 5,000 mg of BCAAs, digestive enzymes and glutamine, along with 20 g of protein, 4 g of carbs, 2 g of fiber and 1 g of fat.

Beyond Your Kitchen Table

Eating is a highly social activity, and enjoying a meal in a nice restaurant can be a real treat. On the other hand, many restaurants are notorious for super-size portions. Often, they will also ease the wait for your meal by offering baskets of white bread and butter. I encourage you to continue enjoying your favorite restaurants, but make sure you stick to your program. Here are some tips to help you make good choices and avoid some of the common pitfalls of eating out.

- Eat a snack before you head out.
- Choose soup or salad as an appetizer.
- Don't feel you have to clear your plate; it is fine if you have to bring half your main dish home.

- Don't be afraid to tweak your meals: ask for the dressing on the side, add protein a salad, remove ingredients or add others.
- Skip the bread.
- Eat two or three appetizers instead of a meal. I do this frequently because it often allows for a grain-free, high-protein meal.

In addition to these basic tips, you may also wish to use these helpful tips that I discovered at the Dietitians Association of Australia:

CUISINE	CHOOSE THESE MORE OFTEN . . .	INSTEAD OF . . .
Bistro	Grilled fish or chicken or steak	Crumbed or fried foods
	Salad bars (choose the salads without dressing and select olive oil and vinegar on the side)	Mixed grill
	Roasted meal of the day	Schnitzels
	Ask for vegetables without butter or heavy sauce	Super-size steak
	Always get vegetables or salad as a side	Creamy sauces like garlic sauce or blue cheese
	Whole-grain bread (or better yet, skip the bread!)	Chips or wedges
		Garlic bread
Mexican	Refried beans	Chimichanga
	Guacamole	Queso fundido (melted cheese)
	Soft taco, burrito or fajita with plenty of salad	Soft taco, burrito or fajita with plenty of sour cream
	Paella	Lots of cheese
	Salsa dip with fresh tortilla	Corn chips (but blue corn chips are lower GI than yellow, so if you have to have some, select these)
Indian	Chicken/prawn masala	Samosa
	Tandoori chicken	Curry puffs
	Dahl	Creamy dishes like korma
	Cucumber raita	Butter chicken
	Roti	Pappadums
	Steamed rice (small portion—no more than $1/2$-cup serving)	Naan bread

CUISINE	CHOOSE THESE MORE OFTEN . . .	INSTEAD OF . . .
Asian	Clear soups	Battered or fried meat dishes like honey chicken
	Braised meat dishes	Dishes made with coconut milk like laksa
	Stir-fried vegetables	Satay dishes
	Chop suey	Fried dim sum or spring rolls
	Nori rolls/sushi	Prawn crackers
	Steamed dim sum	Soy sauce
	Steamed rice (small portion—no more than $1/2$-cup serving)	Fried rice
Italian	Tomato-based sauces like napolitana	Creamy-based sauces like carbonara
	Marinara sauce	Meat-lovers pizzas
	Thin-crust vegetarian pizza; request extra sauce, it makes it so much better!	Pepperoni or salami dishes
	Vegetarian pasta with tomato sauce	Garlic bread
	Pasta with small amount of Parmesan cheese	Pasta with lots of cheese
	Ask for half the cheese on your pizza or request low-fat cheese if possible	Regular cheesy pizza
	Plain bread (better yet, skip the bread!)	Garlic bread with cheese

Source: Adapted from the Dietitians Association of Australia

HORMONE DIET SUCCESS STORY: TINA

"The first day I walked through Dr. Turner's door, I had my lab tests in one hand and a faint glimmer of hope. She assessed my situation and knew immediately that there was an underlying adrenal issue and that my diet, exercise regimen and medication protocol had to change. Years of burning the candle at both ends had compromised the hormonal equivalent of Mother Nature—my adrenals. I was skeptical, but I figured that I had nothing to lose—after all, she has been there herself and knows the perils of a hormonal imbalance. I put her plan in motion, starting with her diet, supplement and exercise recommendations and, lo and behold, I started losing weight! Not only that, but my hair also stopped falling out, my PMS improved and my mood swings diminished.

"Each visit, Dr. Turner would adjust one thing, tweak another, and I would enter the next step of my wellness protocol. I no longer felt like a guinea pig, but an active participant in my own health care. I purchased *The Hormone Diet* and started adding on her other suggestions with great success. While I consider myself to be a 'work in progress,' I know that with *The Hormone Diet* and Dr. Turner's help, I will eventually be the best version of myself, in perfect balance."

TINA

STATS	JUN	MAY	LOST
Weight	126.5	114	12.5
Fat Mass	31.5	21	10.5
Body Fat	24%	19%	5%
BMI	23	20	3

INITIAL CHIEF COMPLAINTS:

1. Hypothyroidism
2. Low adrenals
3. PMS/estrogen dominance
4. Joint and muscle pain

CHAPTER 9

SUPERCHARGED SMOOTHIES

It matters not the number of years in your life.
It is the life in your years.

ABRAHAM LINCOLN

Protein smoothies are not only easy to make but also wonderful for boosting your metabolism. A daily smoothie will provide better appetite control, increased fat burning and blood sugar balance. I have seen these results repeatedly in clinical practice. When you are making your power treat, consider the following super foods or supplements to enhance its therapeutic effects:

1. Whey protein isolate
2. Plain organic yogurt
3. Cinnamon
4. Ground flaxseed
5. Chia seeds
6. Clear fiber
7. L-glutamine powder
8. Inositol

The Foundation: Whey Protein Isolate

When looking for a good whey protein, keep in mind that not all are created equal. I recommend that my patients use a whey protein isolate versus a mixed whey concentrate. While it is a bit more expensive, the benefit of an isolate is that it contains more protein with less fat and lactose per serving. It's a lot easier on the stomach—especially for those who are sensitive to dairy. (See page 105 for more on whey protein isolate.)

A Dollop Will Do: Plain Organic Yogurt

Yogurt is a high water–content food, which means it's a volumizing food that sends the message to your brain that you're full. But, as I mentioned earlier, if you are lactose intolerant or have other sensitivities to dairy, you should leave this one out of your morning smoothie. (See page 108 for more information on plain organic yogurt.)

Sprinkle In: Cinnamon

Cinnamon offers insulin-balancing effects and also seems to reduce several risk factors for cardiovascular disease, including high blood sugar, triglycerides, LDL cholesterol and total cholesterol. Just $^1/_2$ teaspoon a day for 30 days is enough to significantly improve your insulin response *and* trim your waistline. I encourage you to add it to your smoothies and shakes whenever you can. (See page 107 for more information on cinnamon.)

Heaps of: Ground Flaxseed for Cancer Protection

Adding 2 to 3 tablespoons of flaxseed to your smoothies, oatmeal, salads or cereals daily can reduce your cancer risk and also provide a dose of 4 g of fiber and essential fatty acids. As mentioned earlier, be sure to purchase ground flaxseed in a vacuum-sealed package and store in the freezer before it spoils, or grind your own. (See page 99 for more information on ground flaxseed.)

Go for: Ground Chia Seed for Anti-inflammatory Effects

Chia seed is a great addition to a smoothie because it stabilizes blood sugar, manages the effects of diabetes, improves insulin sensitivity and aids symptoms related to metabolic syndrome. It's also a source of omega-3s, fiber, essential amino acids and minerals such as iron, calcium and folic acid. (See page 103 for more information on chia seed.)

Can't Say Enough about Clear Fiber

A wonderful hypoallergenic, non-irritating, psyllium-, corn- and citrus-free fiber, Clear Fiber (Clear Medicine) offers a whopping 8 g of fiber per serving. It is perfect to enhance bowel regularity and to promote healing of the digestive tract wall. The main ingredients are apple fiber, beet fiber, olive oil and vitamin E. Visit drnatashaturner.com to purchase the product. My newest patient recommendation is to use this fiber supplement in smoothies instead of flaxseed or chia seed, which contain only 4 g of fiber per serving. Flaxseed or chia seed can then be sprinkled on another meal to ensure optimal fiber intake.

Soothe and Strengthen: L-Glutamine Powder

L-glutamine is the most abundant amino acid in your body. In times of stress or increased metabolic demand, such as after exercise, it is an especially important nutrient for energy and repair. Glutamine also maintains the health of your intestinal tract and enhances the protective mucosal lining, which helps ensure proper nutrient absorption while limiting the amount of toxins that can pass through your intestinal walls. If you have any form of digestive upset or irritation (such as inflammatory bowel disease, heartburn, reflux, indigestion), L-glutamine can provide a soothing effect.

Balance and Calm: Inositol

Naturally present in many foods, inositol improves the activity of serotonin in the brain. As a supplement, it is an excellent choice for alleviating anxiety, depression and cravings, and for supporting nervous system health. New research suggests this supplement can be helpful for fertility and polycystic ovary syndrome. I add 1 to 2 scoops of a product called Cenitol from Metagenics to my daily smoothie, which gives me about 4 to 12 g of inositol per day.

Smoothie Recipes

Use any of these supercharged recipes for a meal. If you are using one as a snack, reduce the serving size to meet your snack intake requirements. So, instead of 21–30 g of protein, women should have 20 g and men should have 25 g per smoothie. You should also reduce the fruit and milks by half for snack serving sizes. More smoothie recipes can be found in the Recipes section in Part Two.

For each smoothie, place the ingredients in a blender and blend at high speed until smooth.

Berry Bananalicious

1	serving whey protein isolate
2	tablespoons chia seed or ground flaxseed
6	ounces water (or $^1/_2$ cup water and 2 ounces yogurt)
$^1/_3$	cup berry blend
1	small banana (preferably frozen)
4–6	ice cubes

Choco-Bananachino

1	serving whey protein isolate
2	tablespoons chia seed or ground flaxseed or 1 serving of Clear Fiber (Clear Medicine)
2	teaspoons cocoa powder
$^1/_2$	teaspoon cinnamon
4	ounces milk/soy milk/yogurt/almond milk
$^1/_4$	cup water
$^1/_2$	small banana (preferably frozen)
4–6	ice cubes

Banana Berry Power

1	serving whey protein isolate
2	tablespoons chia seed or ground flaxseed or 1 serving Clear Fiber (Clear Medicine)
$^1/_2$	cup milk/soy milk/almond milk
$^1/_4$	cup water
$^1/_2$	cup strawberries (fresh or frozen)
$^1/_2$	banana
4–6	ice cubes

Antioxidant Smoothie

1	serving whey protein isolate
2	tablespoons chia seed or ground flaxseed or 1 serving Clear Fiber (Clear Medicine)
$^1/_2$	cup milk/soy milk/almond milk
$^1/_4$	cup water
$^1/_2$	cup blueberries (fresh or frozen)
1	small banana
4–6	ice cubes

Tasty Tropical Delight

1	serving whey protein isolate
2	tablespoons chia seed or ground flaxseed or 1 serving Clear Fiber (Clear Medicine)
$^1/_4$	cup orange juice
$^1/_2$	cup water
$^1/_2$	cup diced pineapple (fresh or frozen)
$^1/_2$	cup raspberries (fresh or frozen)
4–6	ice cubes

Creamy Creamsicle

- 1 serving whey protein isolate (vanilla)
- 2 tablespoons chia seed or ground flaxseed or 1 serving Clear Fiber (Clear Medicine)
- 1/4 cup orange juice
- 1/2 cup milk/soy milk/almond milk
- 1/2 banana
- 4–6 ice cubes

Cocoa-Coffee Delight

- 1 serving whey protein isolate (vanilla)
- 2 tablespoons chia seed or ground flaxseed or 1 serving Clear Fiber (Clear Medicine)
- 2 tablespoons cocoa powder
- 3 ounces milk/soy milk/almond milk
- 3 ounces coffee
- 4–6 ice cubes

Berry Delicious

- 1 serving whey protein isolate (vanilla)
- 2 tablespoons chia seed or ground flaxseed or 1 serving Clear Fiber (Clear Medicine)
- 3/4 cup water
- 1/3 cup berry blend (fresh or frozen)
- 1/2 banana
- 4–6 ice cubes

Tropical Delight

1	serving whey protein isolate (vanilla)
2	tablespoons chia seed or ground flaxseed or 1 serving Clear Fiber (Clear Medicine)
6	ounces water
$^1/_3$	cup diced pineapple (fresh or frozen)
$^1/_3$	cup diced mango (fresh or frozen)
4–6	ice cubes

Peaches-N-Cream

1	serving whey protein isolate (vanilla)
2	tablespoons chia seed or ground flaxseed or 1 serving Clear Fiber (Clear Medicine)
2	ounces orange juice
4	ounces water
$^3/_4$	cup sliced peaches (fresh or frozen)
$^1/_2$	banana
4–6	ice cubes

Clear Energy Smoothie

1	serving whey protein isolate (vanilla)
2	tablespoons chia seed or ground flaxseed or 1 serving Clear Fiber (Clear Medicine)
$^1/_4$	cup raspberries
$^1/_4$	cup sliced strawberries
$^1/_4$	cup blueberries
$^3/_4$	cup low-fat plain soy milk/almond milk
4	ice cubes

Note: You may use $^3/_4$ cup of fresh or frozen berry blend instead of raspberries, strawberries and blueberries.

Açaí-Avocado Smoothie

- 1 serving whey protein isolate (vanilla)
- 1 tablespoon chia seed or ground flaxseed or 1 serving of Clear Fiber (Clear Medicine)
- 1/4 cup peeled and sliced avocado, frozen
- 1 Sambazon Açaí Smoothie Pack, frozen
- Water to desired consistency

Blueberry-Avocado Smoothie

- 1 serving whey protein isolate (vanilla)
- 1 tablespoon chia seed or ground flaxseed or 1 serving of Clear Fiber (Clear Medicine)
- 3/4 cup blueberries, frozen
- 1/4 cup peeled and sliced avocado, frozen
- Water to desired consistency

Antiaging Smoothie

- 1 serving whey protein isolate (vanilla)
- 2 tablespoons chia seed or ground flaxseed or 1 serving of Clear Fiber (Clear Medicine)
- 1/4 cup raspberries
- 1/4 cup blueberries
- 1/4 cup sliced strawberries
- 1/4 cup blackberries
- 1 cup water

Note: You may use 1 cup of fresh or frozen four-berry blend instead of the berries listed above.

Dopamine Delight Smoothie

- 1 serving whey protein isolate (vanilla)
- 1 tablespoon ground chia seed or ground flaxseed or 1 serving of Clear Fiber (Clear Medicine)
- 1/2 teaspoon ground cinnamon
- 1/2 banana, frozen
- 3/4 cup soy milk (vanilla or plain)/almond milk
- 1 double shot (approx. 1/4 cup) espresso (preferably organic)

Super-satisfying Shake

- 1 serving whey protein isolate (vanilla)
- 2 tablespoons chia seed or ground flaxseed or 1 serving of Clear Fiber (Clear Medicine)
- 1/2 small banana, sliced, or 1/2 cup diced pineapple (fresh or frozen)
- 1/4 cup sliced strawberries (fresh or frozen)
- 1/4 cup sliced mango (fresh or frozen)
- 1 cup water

Serotonin-surge Smoothie

- 1 serving whey protein isolate (vanilla)
- 2 tablespoons chia seed or ground flaxseed or 1 serving of Clear Fiber (Clear Medicine)
- 1 teaspoon cocoa powder
- 1/2 small banana, sliced
- 1 tablespoon almond butter
- 3/4 cup low-fat plain soy milk/almond milk

Testosterone-surge Smoothie

- 1 serving whey protein isolate (vanilla)
- 2 tablespoons ground flaxseed
- 1 cup blueberries (fresh or frozen)
- ½ banana
- 1 cup low-fat plain soy milk/almond milk

"My story is simple. I began suffering with symptoms of *irrational crying episodes*, which alternated with *unbearable irritability*, where I would lash out at the people I cared about the most. And then . . . such dark feelings of *despondency and depression* that I took to my bed and decided to hide from the world.

"After a week and no change I knew I had to do *something*. My family doctor and a referring gynecologist confirmed that menopause was the culprit and offered me antidepressants or hormone replacement therapy. I didn't feel these were the right options for me and so, through a network of friends, I found a naturopath that I hoped would offer me an alternative.

"Enter Dr. Natasha Turner. From the first day I came into her office, I felt hopeful. She listened to my story and confidently told me that she felt certain she could help. She immediately started me on a regimen of bioidentical hormone therapy, dietary supplements after reviewing my blood tests, and she recommended I follow the Hormone Diet.

"I didn't even think of it as a 'diet' . . . but saw it as a new beginning . . . a new lifestyle. And honestly, after the first 3 weeks, I never really found it difficult or felt deprived. I started reading through *The Hormone Diet* and began to have a lot of '*aha*' moments and '*I didn't know that, but it makes sense*' moments. I had no idea so much of our health can be affected by hormones!

"Well, after 10 months and an 87-pound weight loss—I am where I should be . . . I FEEL GREAT! And that's why my horrific menopause was the greatest thing that could have happened to me. It was my 'reason for change' and it brought me to Dr. Turner and the Hormone Diet. The hard part of my story was finding the *right* information to follow; the simple part was following it."

MARLENE, AGE 54

STATS	FEB	JAN	LOST
Weight	215.5	128.5	87
Fat Mass	92.2	28.8	63.4
Body Fat	43%	22%	21%
BP	130/80	120/70	↓

INITIAL CHIEF COMPLAINTS:

1. Menopause
2. Headaches
3. Constipation
4. Depressed, angry, irritable
5. Mood swings, crying

CHAPTER 10

WEEK 5 AND BEYOND:
YES, CHEATING IS REQUIRED!

Anything unattempted remains impossible.

UNKNOWN

By now I am sure you have made some wonderful changes and experienced numerous health improvements. This chapter contains a few tips to help ensure your metabolism and fat-burning hormones are primed—and that they stay that way. I've included additional routines that must be adopted in order to maintain the benefits of your *Supercharged* Hormone Diet plan and to keep you progressing. You will also find some simple solutions to one roadblock: stress! Let's get to it.

Cheat Once a Week

Once you have reached week 5, one of your rules is to incorporate a cheat meal once a week. Your only restriction is that you must not consume any of the foods you are to avoid 100 percent of the time; otherwise all your desires are up for grabs.

Why the cheat meal? Continuous caloric restriction is not an effective long-term fat-loss solution because it is simply not sustainable. The short-term victories achieved with this type of eating are *always* followed by rebound weight gain because, whether we like it or not, hormones will kick in to return the body to its previous state. And, as you will remember from Chapter 2, repeatedly losing and gaining weight is also linked to cardiovascular disease, stroke, diabetes and altered immune function. Therefore, any habit that can prevent yo-yo dieting is a good one to adopt.

From a physiological standpoint, the cheat meal serves to increase your thyroid hormone (particularly the conversion of T4 to T3), to lower levels of Reverse T3 (which can block the action of T3) and to generally boost your metabolism. Remember that the human body is an adaptation machine. When you reduce calories overall, the body adapts and lowers your metabolism as a survival mechanism. Believe it or not, introducing a weekly cheat meal keeps your metabolism guessing and will actually increase your long-term success. It prevents hunger and cravings and refuels your muscles' stores of energy, particularly glycogen, which helps to maintain your strength and endurance for your workouts.

I usually advise my patients to begin incorporating their cheat meal during week 4 or 5 because at this point you have successfully adopted a new way of eating and are closer to achieving your ideal body composition (if you haven't reached it yet). It is important, however, to distinguish this meal from a full-out binge, which will increase insulin levels and decrease fat mobilization. Instead, think of your cheat meal as 1 hour a week where you can let loose a bit, incorporate a treat or dine out without worrying about whether the food will be Hormone Diet–compliant. If we are following the 90/10 principle, where 90 percent of your meals follow the rules outlined in *The Hormone Diet,* then your cheat meal falls into the 10 percent category.

Snacks, Snacks and More Snacks

If you wish to continue having two hormonally balanced smoothies, a day, you certainly are free to do so at this point. If you need alternatives to your smoothies, here are a few quick-and-easy hormonally balanced snack options for you:

1. 2 slices of low-fat Swiss cheese or Jarlsberg cheese
2. 1 to 2 servings of Cabot 75% less fat cheese with a small piece of fruit or a few nuts

3. 1 small organic apple or $^1/_2$ large apple with 1 tablespoon almond butter and 1 slice low-fat cheese
4. 1 serving of plain Greek yogurt with one piece of your permitted fruits
5. 12 almonds and 1 slice of Swiss cheese
6. A Quest Bar (sucrose-free only)
7. $^1/_2$ cup berries mixed with $^1/_2$ cup ricotta cheese
8. 12 tamari-roasted almonds with $^1/_2$ cup blackberries
9. A hard-boiled egg with cucumber slices
10. $^1/_2$ cup hummus with veggie slices (cucumber, peppers, 12 baby carrots)
11. 2 to 3 slices of nitrate- and sulfite-free turkey
12. $^1/_2$ cup low-fat cottage or ricotta cheese mixed with $^1/_4$ cup organic plain or vanilla yogurt
13. Goat milk yogurt with one piece of low-glycemic-index fruit
14. 1 tablespoon pumpkin butter with 2 Wasa or Ryvita Crispbread
15. 2 to 3 tablespoons pumpkin seeds
16. 7 walnuts with a piece of fruit
17. 4 pieces of Ryvita High Fiber Snack Bread, 8 almonds, 1 $^1/_2$ ounces Nu Tofu nonfat Cheddar cheese alternative
18. Mix $^1/_2$ cup organic plain yogurt, $^1/_2$ scoop whey protein isolate, 3 walnuts or 5 almonds and $^1/_4$ cup raspberries or blackberries

Dose up Your Dopamine

Tyrosine is an amino acid—a building block of dopamine and thyroid hormones in the body—and a supplement available at most health-food stores. It takes 4 weeks to reach full effectiveness, so starting this at the beginning of a weight-loss program is a good idea, since studies show levels of dopamine decrease after a few weeks of being on a program to reduce weight. As a brain chemical, dopamine influences pleasure, alertness, learning, creativity, attention and concentration.

Besides the many pleasures dopamine brings, this phenomenal substance naturally suppresses appetite and aids weight loss.

Antidepressant drugs such bupropion (Wellbutrin or Zyban), which act on dopamine receptors in the brain, have been found to help with weight loss. A study at Duke University Medical Center showed weight loss occurred within just a few weeks and remained after a period of 2 years with bupropion use. Many of the study participants who took dopamine also reported feeling satisfied with smaller amounts of foods.

The trouble is, as you lose weight, fat-loss-friendly dopamine tends to take a dip. It's just one of the ways your body works against you by attempting to maintain its regular state of being. But you can wake up your metabolism by supplementing with 1,000 to 3,000 mg of tyrosine each morning on an empty stomach. Seeing as tyrosine increases the production of both dopamine and thyroid hormone, it could give you just the boost you need to push past your plateau. Take 1,000 to 2,000 mg a day of L-tyrosine, away from food. Note: Do not take this supplement if you have high blood pressure or hyperthyroidism.

Strength Training: A Metabolic Must

Gary Taubes is a journalist with the *New York Times*. In his October 2007 article, "The Scientist and the Stairmaster," Taubes suggests, based on over 20 years of research, that exercise does *not* cause weight loss because it stimulates our appetite. As a result, we simply replace the calories we expend through exercise by eating more. In fact, he goes on to recommend *against* exercising and promotes dieting by restricting carbohydrate intake, which leads to less insulin release, as the only effective approach for weight loss.

While eating to limit insulin release is a necessity for fat loss, Taubes fails to consider a significant issue: what about muscle? Dieting does nothing to build the metabolically active muscle we need for optimal fat burning. And what about all the other benefits of exercise? Plenty of research shows that regular workouts boost mood, build bone density, reduce cancer risks, help prevent

Alzheimer's disease, perk up libido and so much more. *Avoiding exercise is not the answer,* no matter how badly we may wish this to be the case. While I do agree that excessive strenuous cardiovascular exercise such as running can actually do more harm than good, a sensible workout program that includes strength training is essential for successful, lasting fat loss. Strength training is the secret that guarantees your metabolism stays revving for the rest of your life. Even more, it helps you keep the weight *off* after you lose it. While the fat on your stomach may seem unattractive, the fat around your organs is more likely to cause disease than surface flab is. But it's easy to keep that visceral fat off, once you lose it.

A new study in the journal *Obesity* found that people who lost weight (including visceral fat) and exercised 80 minutes a week did not regain visceral fat after a year. Those who didn't work out but still kept a healthy weight had 25 percent more visceral fat.

The metabolic equation is very simple: the more muscle tissue you have, the more calories you will burn. Even the process of breaking down and repairing your muscles post-workout increases your metabolism. Miriam Nelson, a Tufts University researcher, showed that a group of women who followed a weight-loss diet *and* did weight-training exercises lost 44 percent more fat than those who only followed the diet. While aerobic activity can help burn calories during the activity, building muscle via strength training means you will continue to burn more calories even while you sleep. And doing your cardio sessions right after your strength training will render even better results. A new study from the College of New Jersey confirms that pumping iron can make your cardio workout more effective. Participants who performed an intense weight workout before riding a stationary bike burned more fat during their cardio session than those who pedaled but skipped the weights. So remember to do your cardio sessions post-workout (never before and not too long).

Now that we know the benefits of strength training and the impact it has on our metabolic rate, what about the impact on our schedule?

The good news is that you won't be spending hours in the gym. In fact, I recommend that all my patients follow a circuit strength-training routine, which is short, intense and no longer than 30 minutes. In order to lose fat, the body must expend more calories than it takes in, but it must also discriminate. High-intensity, short-duration resistance training can provide the needed level of stimulus without placing excessive stress on the recovery system (i.e., your adrenal glands and nervous system). Circuit training is the best type of workout for improving insulin response, boosting testosterone and stimulating growth hormone. Working multiple muscle groups during your workout is also known to boost strength, according to researchers in Canada and Australia. So get your muscles working and spend less time exercising while reaping the most benefit.

Remember that your maintenance exercise prescription includes one or two yoga classes, one or two interval cardio sessions and three strength-training workouts each and every week. The strength-training program, complete with pictures, is clearly outlined in *The Carb Sensitivity Program.* I encourage you to reference this guide, and I promise you that the effects of this workout speak for themselves. I also recommend this book for those wishing to continue weight loss—as it will help you uncover the possible healthy carb options permitted in week 5 and beyond, which can cause hormone disruption and weight gain. Yet another way I help you to personalize and perfect your diet!

TIMING IS EVERYTHING

Cortisol release during exercise appears to depend on the time of day we choose to work out. In 2001, a research team led by Jill Kanaley, Director of the Human Performance Laboratory at Syracuse University, found cortisol was much higher during and after exercise at 7 a.m. than at 7 p.m. or midnight. So, does this mean we shouldn't exercise in the morning if we are under a lot of stress? In this instance, exercise after work or in the early evening might offer us the most stress protection. From a strength perspective, the activation of fast-twitch muscle fibers—which are called into action when force requirements are high—is enhanced at a higher body temperature, which tends to peak in the early evening. If your workouts involve a lot of strength- or power-based movements, chances are you'll perform a little better in the evening than you will in the early morning. So you may want to do your cardio in the morning, since just the right amount can help to reduce cortisol, and your strength training in the evening, when cortisol is lower, to allow for greater muscle growth.

Crank up Your Fat Burning with Interval Cardio Sessions

During week 5 and beyond, you will also move from a moderate-intensity cardio regimen to one complete with interval training for optimal fat burning. An interval is a short burst of exercise performed at a higher intensity for a specific, usually brief, period of time. Each interval is separated from the next by a short rest or lighter activity. To truly benefit from interval training, you must be willing to shake the mindset that endless (and boring!) cardio training is the key to weight loss. Brief, intense bursts of exercise at 80 to 95 percent of your maximum heart rate, interspersed with recovery interludes during which your heart rate returns to normal, burn more calories than steady, less-intense cardio. They also improve performance. For instance, cyclists doubled their endurance after just 2 weeks of sprint-interval training, according to a study in the *Journal of Applied Physiology*. Interval-training principles also apply to running, stair-climbing, rowing and circuits.

For example, 25 minutes of running can be more effective than 40. How? You will burn more fat during and after your workout if you run for 10 minutes at a steady pace, and *then* alternate 1 minute fast and 1 minute slow for the next 10 minutes and run at a slower pace for the last 5 minutes to cool down. Even though you're exercising for a shorter period, you'll still have greater fat loss using this method. And you get to be creative with your cardio routine!

According to another 2001 study conducted at East Tennessee State University, high-intensity interval sessions increase the resting metabolic rate (RMR) for a full 24 hours due to excess post-exercise oxygen consumption (also known as the exercise "after-burn" or the calories expended after an exercise session). This type of exercise may also improve maximum oxygen consumption more effectively than doing only traditional, long aerobic workouts. Alternating intense cardio with moderate cardio is also a great way to expend calories without risking injury. For a complete interval cardio program you can check out the exercise chapter in *The Hormone Diet*.

Keep on Tracking!

According to a study by Wing and Phelan published in the *American Journal of Clinical Nutrition* (2005) about the determinants of success in long-term weight loss, those who lost the weight and kept it off did the following to maintain their success for at least 2 to 5 years after the study:

1. They engaged in high levels of physical activity (approximately 1 hour daily), to maintain their weight loss.
2. They continued to watch their fat and calorie intake.
3. They ate breakfast regularly.
4. They continued to monitor their weight.
5. They maintained a consistent eating pattern across weekdays and weekends.

When you compare these habits with those you have adopted over the past 4 weeks, know that you don't have to count calories, overly restrict your fat intake, exercise an hour a day or skip your cheat meal on the weekend. But I do think it's a good idea to continue weighing yourself daily, or at least once a week, because it will help you to maintain your results. The slim 85-year-olds I have in my office all say the same thing: they weigh themselves daily, and if they are up a pound from one day to the next, they simply skip dessert.

Recognize Stress and Rest Easy

We've talked a lot about the negative effects of stress. But prolonged mental and emotional stresses are particularly injurious because they're usually not followed by a relaxation response the way most physical stress is. As long as the perceived stressful event remains constant in our mind, our body cannot fully achieve a resting, healthy, balanced state. An extended state of imbalance leads to permanent physiological changes over time.

Even worse, we tend to respond to periods of extreme mental and emotional stress with behaviors that serve only to further compromise our health. What do we do when we are faced with tight deadlines, marital difficulties, financial woes or relationship tensions? We stay at work late, eat greasy or sugar-laden foods, drink alcohol, smoke, avoid the gym, fail to sleep enough and skip taking our vitamins just when our body needs healthy habits most.

You must step up your stress-busting strategy, especially if you have stubborn belly fat. The elevated cortisol that comes with stress inhibits thyroid function. As a result, cortisol is indirectly responsible for a lagging metabolism, more water retention and abdominal fat gain. Try meditation, visualization or massage to help keep your cortisol in check. If you are under a lot of stress, consider Relora, or one of the other supplements listed in the next chapter, to lower cortisol.

Relora is my favorite choice for chronic stress and sleep disruption and, boy, does it work! A mixture of the herbal extracts *Magnolia officinalis* and *Phellodendron amurense*, Relora is medically proven to reduce stress and anxiety. It's often the best option for patients who tend to wake up throughout the night, for highly stressed individuals and for menopausal women with hot flashes that cause sleep disruption. It can significantly reduce cortisol and raises DHEA within only 2 weeks of use. Take 2 before bed and 1 in the morning to ease the effects of stress and improve your rest. I recommend Clear Balance—Stress Modifying Formula (Clear Medicine), which contains a mixture of B vitamins and folic acid as well (available through drnatashaturner.com).

Don't forget the importance of sleep for your hormones and metabolism, especially if you find you are struggling to stay on track. Sleep influences the hormones that control your appetite and increase your metabolism. In fact, it's a major regulator of appetite-controlling hormones and also links the extent of hormonal variations with the degree of hunger change. It's no coincidence that insufficient slumber causes you to crave high-calorie, high-sugar foods.

If you need additional remedies to help you improve your sleep, try one or more of these:

Magnesium glycinate—I once had a patient question whether I had given him a drug because this simple mineral worked so well for his sleep! Magnesium calms your nervous system, induces relaxation, reduces blood pressure, decreases cravings, aids PMS tension, increases energy during the day and treats and prevents constipation and muscle cramps. It's truly one of nature's "wonder drugs." Take 200 to 800 mg at night. Keep increasing the dosage until you reach bowel tolerance (the point at which you develop loose stools).

Ashwagandha—Ayurvedic practitioners use this dietary supplement to enhance mental and physical performance, improve learning ability and decrease stress and fatigue. Ashwagandha is a general tonic that can be used in stressful situations, especially for insomnia or restlessness or when you are feeling overworked. Studies have indicated that ashwagandha offers anti-inflammatory, anticancer, antistress, antioxidant, immune-modulating and rejuvenating properties. The typical dosage is 500 to 1,000 mg twice daily. Capsules should be standardized to 1.5 percent with anolides per dose.

GABA—GABA is an inhibitory neurotransmitter, a brain chemical that has a calming effect. It's well suited for individuals who experience anxiety, muscle tension or pain. Take 500 to 1,000 mg before bed. Alternatively, take GABA 10 to 20 minutes before your evening meal for appropriate absorption. The standard dose of 200 mg three times daily can be increased to a maximum of 450 mg three times daily, if needed, but this dosage should not be exceeded. (See Clear Calm—Gaba Enhancing Formula [Clear Medicine] at drnatashaturner.com.)

5-HTP—A derivative of tryptophan that also contributes to the creation of serotonin, 5-HTP has been found to be more effective than tryptophan in treating sleep loss related to depression, anxiety and fibromyalgia. 5-HTP appears to increase REM sleep. It also decreases the amount of time required to fall asleep, as well as the number of nighttime awakenings. Take 50 to 400 mg a day, divided into doses throughout the day or before bed. (See Clear Mood—Serotonin Support Formula [Clear Medicine] at drnatashaturner.com.)

Melatonin—This hormone decreases as we age, as well as during times of stress and depression. Take 0.5 to 3 mg at bedtime. Try opening the capsules and pouring them under your tongue. Better yet, you can also purchase melatonin in sublingual form for fast absorption. Supplements tend to be effective for insomnia only when melatonin levels are low, so if you find it doesn't work for you, this could be the reason. The Xymogen brand of melatonin is my personal favorite.

SEVEN LESSER KNOWN CONSEQUENCES OF A LACK OF SLEEP

While sleep deprivation is likely the last thing on your wish list, you may be surprised to find that it can be the culprit behind some very mysterious symptoms—from increased cravings to skin aging. Here are seven reasons to get your sleep back on track that might surprise you.

IT CAN MAKE YOU LOOK OLDER. One of the first things I notice in my patients after we've restored their sleep patterns is that they look remarkably younger—and now science backs this observation. Researchers at University Hospitals (UH) Case Medical Center demonstrated that poor sleepers had increased signs of skin aging and slower recovery from a variety of environmental stressors, such as disruption of the skin barrier or ultraviolet (UV) radiation. They also had a worse assessment of their own skin and facial appearance. This quick-trip to aging is likely from the reduced growth hormone and increased cortisol levels that go hand-in-hand with a sleepless night. It turns out that sleep is the foundation of youth, after all.

YOU'LL WANT MORE HIGH-CALORIE SNACKS. It's no surprise that those sleepless nights will send your appetite to a bad place and a 2013 UC Berkeley study confirms it's for calorie-dense junk food like burgers, potato chips and sweets. Using an MRI machine, researchers scanned the brains of 23 healthy young adults, first after a normal night's sleep and next, after a sleepless night. They found impaired activity in the sleep-deprived brain's frontal lobe, which governs complex decision-making but increased activity in deeper brain centers that respond to rewards. In other words, the participants favored junk food the day after a restless night. Case in point, you can't get to your weight loss goals without looking at your sleeping habits.

YOU AND YOUR SPOUSE WILL FIGHT MORE. Scientists have learned that a lack of sleep can cause relationship issues. Not to mention that relationship issues can cause a lack of sleep, so be careful not to fall into this cycle. UC Berkeley psychologists Amie Gordon and Serena Chen discovered that couples were more likely to argue and engage in unnecessary conflict after a bad night's sleep. So not only should you not go to bed angry, you may find your relationship improves when you get your 7 to 8 hours of sleep a night.

YOU'LL FEEL MORE ACHES AND PAINS. A lack of sleep can impair your natural pain control mechanisms and exacerbate those nagging aches and pains, according to results of a 2011 study published in *Arthritis & Rheumatism*. Researchers from Norway have uncovered an association between sleep problems and increased risk of fibromyalgia in women. The opposite is also true—extending your sleep can reduce your pain sensitivity. In fact, for those who suffer from migraines, a good night's sleep may be your first defense.

IT CAN AFFECT YOUR DATING LIFE. Chances are you've heard the term "beer goggles," but researchers at Hendrix College in Arkansas found that "insomnia goggles" may have a similar effect. The study showed that among college men it can affect their judgment in romantic situations—more specifically the frontal lobe's reign over inhibition and moral reasoning. If you want to get an accurate vibe on whether or not your date is really interested in you, be sure you get between 7 and 8 hours of sleep the night before.

YOUR ANXIETY WILL GET WORSE. Whether or not you're prone to anxiety, a few nights without proper sleep can transform you into an excessive worrier. Neuroscientists, again from UC Berkeley, found that sleep deprivation amplifies anticipatory anxiety by affecting regions associated with emotional processing. If your mood is low and your anxiety is high, consider the most natural antidepressant around—sleep therapy.

YOUR INSULIN-SENSITIVITY WILL BE REDUCED. Your instinct to hit the snooze button may be right. Researchers from the University of Pittsburgh discovered that teens who normally get 6 hours of sleep per night can improve their insulin resistance by 9 percent by adding 1 extra hour of sleep. It seems like a simple solution to the belly fat problem, although it does take practice. A ritual for getting sleep should begin a few hours before bed, versus in the 15 minutes before. Try turning off all bright devices (yes, this includes cell phones and laptops) and install a dimmer that you flick on in the evenings to allow yourself to wind down. During the weeks when our schedules get the best of us, use the weekends to catch up on those lost hours—and reduce your risk of type 2 diabetes.

Feel the Heat: Body Temperature and Appetite

Beyond the caloric expenditure involved in maintaining a constant core temperature, heat can help to control our weight by suppressing our appetite. An all-you-can-eat buffet certainly loses its appeal when we're hot. But people living with constant climate control often fail to feel the heat. Now don't go cranking up your thermostat just yet! Heat does not work for long-term weight control because it tends to decrease our basal metabolic rate. When we're constantly warm, less thyroid hormone is required to generate heat via our metabolism.

As we age, our natural ability to maintain and control our body temperature becomes less reliable. Our temperature also closely affects our sleep quality because we need to cool down slightly in order to properly activate the release of sleep-enhancing melatonin. We also know that sleep quality directly influences our body composition. Could poor temperature control be yet another reason for weight gain and hormonal imbalance as we age? I think so.

When it comes to sleep, the vast majority of my patients report experiencing far more restful nights after they get started on the Hormone Diet. I have always thought these improvements were brought about by consistently balancing blood sugar, which helps to stabilize stress hormones (remember, skipped and unbalanced meals raise cortisol). I am still certain that blood sugar balance plays a role, but I have also found a study in the *Journal of Biorhythms* (2002) that links melatonin production to the carbohydrate content of evening meals. After only 3 days of consuming carbohydrate-rich meals in the evening, salivary melatonin levels were reduced in otherwise healthy men. Less melatonin release, as we know, can cause sleep disruption.

Without realizing it, I was encouraging better melatonin release in my patients by recommending that they avoid excessive carb consumption at dinner. What's the link? Body temperature rises when we eat too many carbohydrates and stays elevated for about 8 hours after consumption. The warmer we are, the less melatonin is released during sleep.

Alcohol also increases our nighttime temperature, which could be another reason for its sleep-disrupting effects, besides its impact on our blood sugar and stress hormones. Researchers from France suggest this may also explain some clinical signs observed in alcoholic patients, including sleep and mood disorders. The researchers went on to say that the negative effects of jet lag, shift work and aging—all of which are known to alter our body temperature by influencing our hormones—can be aggravated by alcohol. These factors can, therefore, affect our waistline too.

At the same time, sleep deprivation makes us colder because it lowers both our metabolic rate and our thyroid hormones. As I have already explained, when we feel colder, we feel hungrier, and we eat more. Clearly, sleep deprivation and temperature changes are a double whammy when it comes to overeating and weight gain. I wonder what would happen if we made the effort to stay extra warm on the days we are sleep deprived. Would we still consume as many calories and sweets? Fascinating questions like these are one of the reasons I love hormones so much. Nothing occurs in isolation when it comes to hormones.

HOT ON HORMONAL HEALTH
HOW YOUR BODY TEMPERATURE AFFECTS YOUR HORMONES, METABOLISM AND APPETITE

Ahhh, that climate control. We certainly spend a lot of money and energy trying to keep ourselves at a comfortable temperature. But in doing so, we create a situation in which our bodies expend less energy in the form of calories. In the end, all the cool comfort may be making us fatter!

Every day, we burn a certain amount of energy just maintaining our internal equilibrium, including our body temperature. Energy comes in by way of food and is expended through activities such as working, exercising and even the passive activities such as body temperature regulation, breathing, the pumping of our heart and all sorts of vital stuff. According to the old weight-loss formula, we lose pounds when we burn more calories than we take in. But if we take away the caloric expenditure needed to maintain our temperature, the unused calories will end up somewhere, usually in the form of fat.

Hard to believe, I know, but climate control can make us fatter. In a study published in the *International Journal of Obesity* (June 2006), University of Alabama at Birmingham biostatistician Dr. David Allison suggested that air conditioning is one of 10 factors that may play an important role in today's weight crisis. Dr. Allison showed a fascinating link between the huge proliferation of air conditioning in the southern United States and the higher prevalence of obesity in this region.

Changes in temperature, either up or down, can be perceived by your body as a stressor to which it must respond. This response requires energy and also influences our hormonal balance. For instance, when our body temperature drops, our sympathetic nervous system releases adrenaline, our blood vessels constrict to prevent heat loss (good for keeping us warm, not great for a glowing complexion in the long run) and we may also start to shiver. When we are hot, more blood flow is directed toward our skin to allow heat to radiate into our surroundings. Sympathetic stimulation causes us to start sweating, which also requires calories. In fact, one study showed that women who lived in a constant 80-degree climate burned almost 250 more calories per day at rest than women in a 70-degree environment.

Your Macronutrient Makeup Moving Forward

During the past 4 weeks, you have been consuming meals that are slightly higher in protein simply for its powerful hormonal and metabolic benefits. Now that you have woken up your metabolism, you can move forward, eating meals that are slightly higher in lower-glycemic carbohydrates. All of the recipes in *The Hormone Diet* meet these criteria. So, along with the strength-training program, you can use any of the more than 70 recipes presented there to enjoy delicious meals and keep your weight maintenance goals on track.

Your Nutrition and Hormone Health Habits Checklist: A Summary

These statements should describe your behaviors at least 90 percent of the time.

- ☐ I record all of my habits on my daily wellness tracker.
- ☐ I eat 2 low-glycemic fruits per day (at least 1 serving of berries daily).
- ☐ I eat organic food whenever possible.
- ☐ I eat 6 or more servings of *non-starchy* vegetables daily.
- ☐ I always avoid soft drinks (diet and regular).
- ☐ I avoid refined (white) carbohydrates and added sugar, except for during my cheat meal.
- ☐ I eat protein at every meal, the size and width of my palm or the suggested serving size on my protein-source food list.
- ☐ I choose low-glycemic whole-food carbohydrates such as quinoa, sweet potatoes and winter squash and consume them in limited amounts (once a day, preferably at lunch or dinner).
- ☐ Stevia and xylitol are the only sweeteners I use; I avoid artificial sweeteners 100 percent of the time.
- ☐ I drink 8 or more glasses of reverse-osmosis water daily.
- ☐ I limit alcohol to no more than 3 glasses of wine (preferably red) weekly.
- ☐ At minimum, I take a multivitamin, vitamin D and omega-3 supplement daily.
- ☐ I avoid high-fructose corn syrup 100 percent of the time.

- ☐ I avoid partially hydrogenated oils and unhealthy inflammatory oils 100 percent of the time.
- ☐ I eat 1 to 2 servings of raw nuts, nut butters and/or seeds daily.
- ☐ I consume 1 serving of extra-virgin olive oil daily.
- ☐ I carry one healthy snack with me all the time to avoid skipped meals, unhealthy snacks and cheating.
- ☐ I avoid microwaving my food and charbroiling my meat.
- ☐ I eat every 3 to 4 hours.
- ☐ I eat within 1 hour of waking.
- ☐ I consume 30 g or more of fiber a day.
- ☐ I stop eating 3 hours before going to bed.
- ☐ I have an afternoon snack containing protein each day.
- ☐ I have 1 serving of whey protein isolate daily.
- ☐ I eat at the same times daily because my body likes routine (e.g., 8 a.m., 12 p.m., 4 p.m. and 7 p.m.).
- ☐ I have a cheat meal once a week to maintain my metabolic rate and healthy thyroid hormone levels.
- ☐ I floss my teeth daily and maintain great oral hygiene.
- ☐ I follow the rules for hormone-enhancing sleep.
- ☐ I manage stress through monthly massage or relaxation techniques such as breathing exercises, meditation or visualization.
- ☐ I complete 3 days of strength training, 1 to 2 days of cardio and 1 to 2 days of yoga each week.
- ☐ I complete my blood tests annually with my doctor.
- ☐ I pay attention to the symptoms my body is trying to show me.
- ☐ I pay attention to the hormone-disrupting ingredients in my skin care products, cleaning products and foods.
- ☐ I complete the *Supercharged* Hormone Diet detox at least once a year to maintain a healthy digestive system, liver function and hormonal balance.

Here's your summary of your daily Glyci-Med food selections:

- 4 equal-size servings of protein
- 3 protein meals and 2 half-servings for snacks (including preferably 1 whey protein and 2 others the size and width of your palm)
- 3 fats (including 1 serving of extra-virgin olive oil daily)
- 2 to 3 fruits (including 1 serving of berries daily)
- 1 starchy carb (about $^1/_2$ cup or the size of your fist)
- 1 to 2 servings of nuts (see recommended serving size in Part Two)
- Unlimited non-starchy veggies (at least 5 or 6 servings)
- Remember, your meals should comprise 35 percent carbohydrate; 35 percent protein and 30 percent fat. Memorize your protein, fat and carb intake guidelines as outlined on pages 116–17.

"I've always struggled with weight loss and unwanted fat through no fault of my own. I say this because I've maintained a fairly healthy lifestyle with diet and exercise, always trying to improve year after year through reading and slowly tweaking what I hope would provide the answer. Then one day on talk radio I heard Dr. Turner and it all made so much sense. I bought her book right away and read it, I think three times, maybe more. I didn't want to miss anything.

"I could relate to so many things she explained in the book. I was ready for the next phase to bring it all together. It really felt like finding the 'ruby in the rubble.' I am now running down that road to health. It's great when pants that were tight are now falling off and you run out of holes on your belt! You wake up feeling slim and it stays with you all day now. No more late-day bloating. My energy is better, skin improved, digestive track is in great shape and finally the fat is coming off in those unwanted areas. Thanks to the Hormone Diet!"

MIKE

STATS	APR	MAY	LOST
Weight	237	230	7
Fat Mass	57.1	52	5.1
Body Fat	24%	22%	2%
BP	139/92	120/80	↓
Waist (inches)	41.5	39	2.5
Hips (inches)	44.5	43	1.5

INITIAL CHIEF COMPLAINTS:

1. Upper body fat
2. Leg cramps
3. Muscle tension
4. Low libido

CHAPTER 11

CREATING YOUR OWN HORMONAL HEALTH PRESCRIPTION

Only those who dare to fail greatly can ever achieve greatly.

ROBERT F. KENNEDY

Now that you have completed your detox, uncovered your food sensitivities and mastered the rules of hormonally balanced nutrition, you've reached the point where you can personalize your own plan. Because everyone completes the same detox and follows the same basic rules for hormonally balanced nutrition, it makes much better sense to individualize your program after you have completed these steps. Tailoring for your specific needs and goals will help to ensure you continue to address any hormonal symptoms that linger after your work thus far.

Within the following pages, you will find a series of checklists of symptoms and conditions. Each checklist pertains to a specific hormonal imbalance or condition that can, in one way or another, impede your weight loss and amplify the negative effects of aging.

As you go through the lists, check off all the symptoms and signs you are currently experiencing within each group. Add up your total for each group and record it in the box provided at the bottom of the list.

Since more than one hormone can cause similar symptoms, you will find a lot of repetition among the different groups. Just keep going, and do your best to be consistent with your answers throughout the entire profile. Doing so will definitely provide you with the most complete picture of your current state of hormonal wellness.

Don't worry if you discover that you still have imbalances

remaining at this stage of your program. Many people find that their symptoms begin to clear within the first 4 weeks. And I will help you to address any symptoms that remain at the end of your *Supercharged* Plan with specific supplements and foods, and the tools I have created in this chapter.

This profile is an exciting, interactive feature of the *Supercharged* Hormone Diet. With your answers in hand, you will be able to fine-tune your hormonal health prescription by adding in specific foods and supplements that address your unique hormone-balancing needs.

Your Hormonal Health Profile

Check off all that apply to you and total your scores in each group.

CONDITION: INFLAMMATION	
Sagging, thinning skin or wrinkling	✓
Spider veins or varicose veins	
Cellulite	
Eczema, skin rashes, hives or acne	
Menopause (women); andropause (men)	
Heart disease	
Prostate enlargement (prostatitis)	
High cholesterol or blood pressure	✓
Loss of muscle tone in arms and legs; difficulty building or maintaining muscle	
Aches and pains	
Arthritis, bursitis, tendonitis or joint stiffness	✓
Water retention in hands or feet	
Gout	
Alzheimer's disease	
Parkinson's disease	
Depression	
Night eating syndrome (waking at night to binge eat)	
Fibromyalgia	
Increased pain or poor pain tolerance	

CONDITION: INFLAMMATION (continued)	
Headaches or migraines	
High alcohol consumption (> 4 drinks per week for women and > 7 drinks per week for men)	
Bronchitis; allergies (food or environmental); hives or asthma have worsened or developed	
Autoimmune disease (lupus, rheumatoid arthritis, etc.)	
Fat gain around "love handles" or abdomen	
Loss of bone density or osteoporosis	
Generalized overweight/weight gain/obesity	
Fatty liver (diagnosed by your doctor)	
Diabetes (type 2)	
Sleep disruptions or deprivation	
Alternating diarrhea and constipation (irritable bowel or inflammatory bowel disease)	
Frequent gas and bloating	
Constipation, diarrhea or nausea	
TOTAL (Warning score: > 11)	

HORMONAL IMBALANCE 1: EXCESS INSULIN	
Age spots and wrinkling	
Sagging skin	
Cellulite	
Skin tags	
Acanthosis nigricans (a skin condition characterized by light brown to black patches or markings on the neck or underarm)	
Abnormal hair growth on face, chin (women)	
Vision changes or cataracts	
Infertility or irregular menses	
Shrinking or sagging breasts	
Menopause (women); andropause or erectile dysfunction (men)	
Heart disease	
High cholesterol, high triglycerides or high blood pressure	

HORMONAL IMBALANCE 1: EXCESS INSULIN (continued)	
Burning feet at night (especially while in bed)	
Water retention in the face/puffiness	
Gout	
Poor memory, concentration, or Alzheimer's disease	
Fat gain around "love handles" and/or abdomen	
Fat over the triceps	
Generalized overweight/weight gain/obesity	
Hypoglycemia; craving for sweets, carbohydrates, or constant hunger or increased appetite	
Fatigue after eating (especially carbohydrates)	
Fatty liver (diagnosed by your doctor)	
Diabetes (type 2)	
Sleep disruption or deprivation	
TOTAL (Warning score: > 9)	

HORMONAL IMBALANCE 2: LOW DOPAMINE	
Fatigue, especially in the morning	
Poor tolerance for exercise	
Restless leg syndrome	
Poor memory	
Parkinson's disease	
Depression	
Loss of libido	
Feeling a strong need for stimulation or excitement (foods, gambling, partying, sex, etc.)	
Addictive eating or binge eating	
Cravings for sweets, carbohydrates, junk food or fast food	
TOTAL (Warning score: > 4)	

HORMONAL IMBALANCE 3: LOW SEROTONIN	
PMS characterized by hypoglycemia, sugar cravings and/or depression	
Feeling wired at night	
Lack of sweating	

HORMONAL IMBALANCE 3: LOW SEROTONIN (continued)	
Poor memory	
Loss of libido	﹨
Depression, anxiety, irritability or seasonal affective disorder	⌐
Loss of motivation or competitive edge	﹗
Low self-esteem	﹒
Inability to make decisions	
Obsessive-compulsive disorder	
Bulimia or binge eating	
Fibromyalgia	
Increased pain or poor pain tolerance	
Headaches or migraines	
Cravings for sweets or carbohydrates	ﹾ
Constant hunger or increased appetite	
Inability to sleep in no matter how late going to bed	
Less than 7.5 hours of sleep per night	﹗
Irritable bowel	
Constipation	
Nausea	
Use of corticosteroids	
TOTAL (Warning score: > 4)	

HORMONAL IMBALANCE 4: LOW GABA	
PMS characterized by breast tenderness, water retention, bloating, anxiety, sleep disruptions or headaches	
Feeling wired at night	
Aches and pains or increased muscle tension	
Irritability, tension or anxiety	
Difficulty falling asleep	
Less than 7.5 hours of sleep per night	
Irritable bowel	
Frequent gas and bloating	
TOTAL (Warning score: > 3)	

HORMONAL IMBALANCE 5: EXCESS CORTISOL

Wrinkling, thinning skin or skin has lost its fullness	
Hair loss	
Infertility or absent menses (unrelated to menopause)	
Feeling wired at night	
Heart palpitations	
Loss of muscle tone in arms and legs	
Cold hands or feet	
Water retention in face/puffiness	
Poor memory or concentration	
Loss of libido	
Depression, anxiety, irritability or seasonal affective disorder	
High alcohol consumption	
Frequent colds and flus	
Hives, bronchitis, allergies (food or environmental), asthma or autoimmune disease	
Fat gain around "love handles" or abdomen	
A "buffalo hump" of fat on back of neck/upper back	
Difficulty building or maintaining muscle	
Loss of bone density or osteoporosis	
Cravings for sweets or carbs, hypoglycemia or constant hunger	
Difficulty falling asleep	
Difficulty staying asleep (especially waking between 2 and 4 a.m.)	
Less than 7.5 hours of sleep per night	
Irritable bowel or frequent gas and bloating	
Use of corticosteroids	
TOTAL (Warning score: > 8)	

HORMONAL IMBALANCE 6: LOW CORTISOL

Feeling "burned out," or fatigued especially in the morning	
Poor tolerance for exercise	
Decreased ability to deal with stress	

HORMONAL IMBALANCE 6: LOW CORTISOL (continued)	
Loss of muscle tone in arms and legs; muscle weakness	
General aches and pains	
Arthritis, bursitis, tendonitis, joint stiffness	
Poor memory	
Loss of motivation or competitive edge	
Increased pain or poor pain tolerance	
Hives, bronchitis, worsened allergies (food or environmental) or asthma	
Loss of libido	
Alternating diarrhea and constipation (or irritable bowel syndrome)	
PMS	
Depression	
Autoimmune disease	
Hypoglycemia	
Low blood pressure or dizziness when moving from sitting or lying to standing	
Cravings for salty foods	
TOTAL (Warning score: > 6)	

HORMONAL IMBALANCE 7: LOW DHEA	
Dry skin	
Heart disease	
Erectile dysfunction	
Andropause	
Feeling wired at night	
Poor tolerance for exercise	
Loss of muscle tone in arms and legs	
Poor memory or concentration	
Irritability or easily agitated	
Loss of libido	
Depression	
Loss of motivation or competitive edge	
Autoimmune disease	

HORMONAL IMBALANCE 7: LOW DHEA (continued)

Fat gain around "love handles"	
Fat gain over the triceps	
Fat gain around the abdomen	
Difficulty building or maintaining muscle	
TOTAL (Warning score: > 6)	

HORMONAL IMBALANCE 8: EXCESS ESTROGEN

Spider or varicose veins	
Cellulite	
Heavy menstrual bleeding	
PMS characterized by breast tenderness, water retention, bloating, swelling and/or weight gain	
Fibrocystic breast disease	
Prostate enlargement	
Erectile dysfunction	
Breast growth (men)	
Loss of morning erection	
Irritability, mood swings or anxiety	
Headaches or migraines (especially in women before their menses)	
High alcohol consumption	
Autoimmune disease or allergies	
Fat gain around "love handles" or abdomen (men)	
Fat gain at the hips (women)	
Current use of hormone replacement therapy or birth control pills	
TOTAL (Warning score: > 6)	

HORMONAL IMBALANCE 9: LOW ESTROGEN

Dry or sagging skin	
Thinning skin or skin has lost its fullness	
Hair loss	
Dry eyes or cataracts (women)	

HORMONAL IMBALANCE 9: LOW ESTROGEN (continued)

PMS characterized by depression, hypoglycemia, sugar cravings and/or sweet cravings	
Infertility or absent menses (not related to menopause)	
Painful intercourse and/or vaginal dryness	
Shrinking or sagging breasts	
Urinary incontinence (stress or otherwise)	
Menopause	
Fatigue	
Hot flashes	
Poor memory or concentration	
Irritability	
Loss of libido	
Depression or mood swings	
Fat gain around "love handles" or abdomen (menopausal women)	
Loss of bone density or osteoporosis	
Difficulty falling or staying asleep	
TOTAL (Warning score: > 8)	

HORMONAL IMBALANCE 10: LOW PROGESTERONE

Dry skin or skin that has lost its fullness	
Spider or varicose veins	
Hair loss	
Short menstrual cycle (< 28 days) or excessively long bleeding times (> 6 days)	
PMS characterized by breast tenderness, anxiety, sleep disruptions, headaches, menstrual spotting, water retention, bloating and/or weight gain	
Infertility or absent menses (not related to menopause)	
Fibrocystic breast disease	
Menopause (women); andropause (men)	
Prostate enlargement	
Hot flashes	
Lack of sweating	
Feeling cold and/or cold hands and feet	

HORMONAL IMBALANCE 10: LOW PROGESTERONE (continued)

Heart palpitations	
Water retention	
Irritability and/or anxiety	
Loss of libido	
Headaches or migraines	
Autoimmune disease, hives, asthma or allergies	
Loss of bone density or osteoporosis	
Difficulty falling or staying asleep	
TOTAL (Warning score: > 6)	

HORMONAL IMBALANCE 11: EXCESS PROGESTERONE

Acne	
PMS characterized by depression	
Infertility	
Water retention	
Depression	
Frequent colds and flus	
Weight gain or difficulty losing weight	
Current use of hormone replacement therapy or birth control pills	
TOTAL (Warning score: > 4)	

HORMONAL IMBALANCE 12: LOW TESTOSTERONE

Dry skin	
Thinning skin or skin has lost its fullness	
Painful intercourse	
Heart diseases (men)	
Erectile dysfunction	
Andropause (men)	
Loss of morning erection	
Fatigue	

HORMONAL IMBALANCE 12: LOW TESTOSTERONE (continued)

Poor tolerance for exercise	
Loss of muscle tone in arms and legs	
Poor memory or concentration	
Loss of libido	
Depression or anxiety	
Loss of motivation or competitive edge	
Headaches or migraines (men)	
Gaining fat around abdomen or "love handles" (men and women)	
Difficulty building or maintaining muscle	
Loss of bone density or osteoporosis (men and women)	
Sleep apnea (men)	
Use of corticosteroids	
TOTAL (Warning score: > 7)	

HORMONAL IMBALANCE 13: EXCESS TESTOSTERONE

Acne	
Acanthosis nigricans (women)	
Hair loss (scalp)	
Abnormal hair growth on face (women)	
Infertility	
Shrinking or sagging breasts	
Prostate enlargement	
Irritability, aggression or easily agitated	
Fat gain at abdomen (women)	
Cravings for sweets or carbohydrates (women)	
Constant hunger or increased appetite (women)	
Fatty liver (women)	
TOTAL (Warning score: > 4)	

HORMONAL IMBALANCE 14: LOW THYROID

Dry skin and/or hair	✓
Acne	
Hair loss	
Brittle hair and/or nails	
PMS, infertility, long menstrual cycle (> 30 days or irregular periods)	
Abnormal lactation	
Fatigue	
Lack of sweating, feeling cold or cold hands and feet	✓
High cholesterol	✓
Poor tolerance for exercise	
Heart palpitations	
Outer edge of eyebrows thinning	✓
Aches and pains	
Water retention/puffiness in hands or feet	
Poor memory	
Loss of libido	
Depression	
Loss of motivation or competitive edge	
Iron deficiency anemia	
Hives	
Generalized overweight/weight gain/obesity	
Constipation	
Use of corticosteroids	
Current use of synthetic hormone replacement or birth control pills	
TOTAL (Warning score: > 8)	

HORMONAL IMBALANCE 15: LOW ACETYLCHOLINE

Poor tolerance for exercise	✓
Loss of muscle tone in arms and legs or poor muscle function/strength	
Poor memory or concentration, decrease in memory or recall	

HORMONAL IMBALANCE 15: LOW ACETYLCHOLINE (continued)

Alzheimer's disease	
Difficulty building or maintaining muscle	
Difficulty falling asleep or staying asleep, disrupted sleep patterns	
Irritable bowel	
Constipation	
TOTAL (Warning score: > 3)	

HORMONAL IMBALANCE 16: LOW MELATONIN

Andropause (men)	
Night eating syndrome	
High alcohol consumption	
Cravings for sweets or carbohydrates; increased appetite	
Difficulty falling asleep	
Failing to sleep in total darkness	
Difficulty staying asleep (especially waking between 2 and 4 a.m.)	
Sleep apnea	
Less than 7.5 hours of sleep per night	
Use of corticosteroids	
TOTAL (Warning score: > 3)	

HORMONAL IMBALANCE 17: LOW GROWTH HORMONE

Dry skin	
Thinning skin or skin has lost its fullness	
Sagging skin	
Menopause (women); andropause (men)	
Lack of exercise	
Loss of muscle tone in arms or legs	
High alcohol consumption	
Fat gain around "love handles" or abdomen	
Difficulty building or maintaining muscle	
Loss of bone density or osteoporosis	

Generalized overweight/weight gain/obesity	
Failing to sleep in total darkness	
Difficulty staying asleep (especially waking between 2 and 4 a.m.)	
Sleep apnea	
Use of corticosteroids	
TOTAL (Warning score: > 5)	

Create Your Own Treatment Pyramid

After you have completed the profile, go ahead and transfer your scores from each group to the appropriate space in the treatment pyramid on the next page.

Use Your Hormonal Health Profile Results to Create Your Personalized Prescription For Hormonal Balance

If your profile revealed *only* one high score, go ahead and address it now with one or more of the options listed on pages 188–216 for the associated hormonal imbalance.

If you have *more than one* high score, start with whichever one appears lowest on the treatment pyramid and work your way up to the highest. You will work your way up to the highest-level imbalance over time. This method is important because correcting a lower-level imbalance may be enough to correct or improve other imbalances noted in the levels above. For example, look at your score in Level 1. If it is high, address it now with one or more of the product recommendations listed on pages 188–216. If you do not have a high score in Level 1, move up to Level 2 or keep going up until you reach the next level with a high score. Each level of the treatment pyramid builds upon the next, which means that besides starting from the bottom, *you should also address imbalances within the same level at the same time.*

As an aside, taking *all* the supplements I have listed for each hormonal imbalance is neither needed nor recommended. Carefully

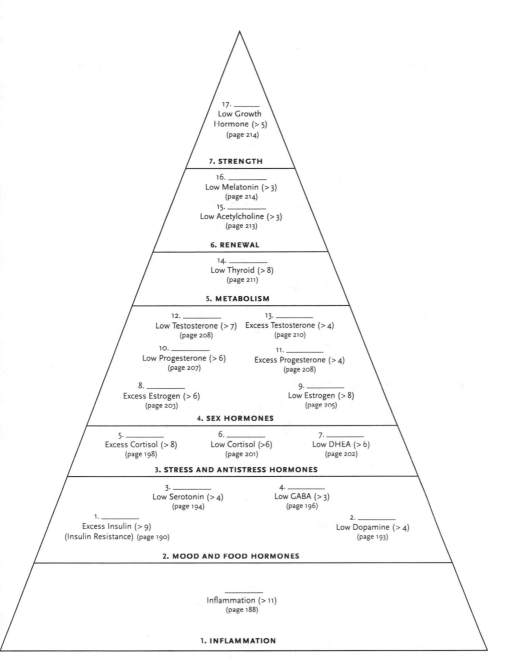

17. _____
Low Growth
Hormone (> 5)
(page 214)

7. STRENGTH

16. _____
Low Melatonin (> 3)
(page 214)

15. _____
Low Acetylcholine (> 3)
(page 213)

6. RENEWAL

14. _____
Low Thyroid (> 8)
(page 211)

5. METABOLISM

12. _____   13. _____
Low Testosterone (> 7)   Excess Testosterone (> 4)
(page 208)   (page 210)

10. _____   11. _____
Low Progesterone (> 6)   Excess Progesterone (> 4)
(page 207)   (page 208)

8. _____   9. _____
Excess Estrogen (> 6)   Low Estrogen (> 8)
(page 203)   (page 205)

4. SEX HORMONES

5. _____   6. _____   7. _____
Excess Cortisol (> 8)   Low Cortisol (>6)   Low DHEA (> 6)
(page 198)   (page 201)   (page 202)

3. STRESS AND ANTISTRESS HORMONES

3. _____   4. _____
Low Serotonin (> 4)   Low GABA (> 3)
(page 194)   (page 196)

1. _____   2. _____
Excess Insulin (> 9)   Low Dopamine (> 4)
(Insulin Resistance) (page 190)   (page 193)

2. MOOD AND FOOD HORMONES

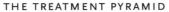
Inflammation (> 11)
(page 188)

1. INFLAMMATION

THE TREATMENT PYRAMID

read the information about each product and choose the supplement you feel suits you the best. Visit drnatashaturner.com for additional product sources and brand recommendations.

How Long Should You Use a Certain Supplement?

You should stick with the treatment suggestions or supplements for each specific imbalance until you feel your symptoms have improved. The severity and duration of the imbalance and, of course, your body's response to the steps will determine the length of time each imbalance requires treatment.

When you feel you are ready, you can return to the pyramid and find your next highest score. Go back and look at the associated group of questions in your profile to identify whether this hormone is still a concern for you. If it is, carry on with the specific treatment suggestions for that hormonal imbalance noted in this chapter.

Don't be surprised if, when you do go back to your profile, symptoms you once had have cleared up. Remember, as you work your way up the pyramid, each level of hormones helps to restore the next.

Keep going through all the levels of the pyramid until you have addressed all of your imbalances. After this point, I recommend revisiting the profile at least once a year to ensure that you're remaining balanced.

Level One Treatment
Condition: Inflammation

Reducing inflammation is absolutely vital to allow the body to lose unwanted fat. Anti-inflammatory supplements help to optimize the fat-burning capabilities of our liver and muscle cells and can also help to reduce the uncomfortable signs and symptoms of inflammation.

SUPPLEMENT OPTIONS:

   1. **Curcumin (Turmeric):** Turmeric has anti-inflammatory, antioxidant, antiaging, immune-enhancing and hormone-balancing

effects. It works as a natural COX-2 inhibitor to cut inflammation, pain and swelling. Turmeric also supports liver function and detoxification. Take 500 to 1,500 mg a day, away from food. In addition, I have Clear Detox—Hormonal Health (Clear Medicine), which contains turmeric, green tea and several other anti-inflammatory ingredients that I find in my clinical practice to be very effective for reducing blood inflammatory markers when patients use a dose of one pack a day for a few months.

2. **Wobenzym:** Wobenzym is the most researched systemic anti-inflammatory enzyme formulation in the world. It is used by Olympic athletes, doctors and millions of Europeans to help normalize all types of inflammation, speed injury recovery, promote healthy aging, aid surgery recovery, relieve arthritis and tendonitis and improve circulation. Wobenzym contains bromelain and other enzymes in enteric-coated tablets that pass through your digestive tract and allow the enzymes to enter your bloodstream. The enzymes are distributed throughout the body along with nutrients and oxygen to benefit all your tissues and organs by breaking down inflammatory proteins. Wobenzym rids the blood of these harmful proteins that can damage joints, blood vessels and other tissues. Take 2 tablets two to three times a day, away from food. This can be increased to 4 to 5 tablets taken two to three times daily during acute inflammatory conditions, post-surgery or to reduce thyroid antibodies.

3. **Nattokinase:** This enzyme is a by-product of the fermentation of soy. It reduces inflammation and aids circulation. I use it specifically for elevated high-sensitivity C-reactive protein (hs-CRP). Take 38 to 50 mg twice a day away from food for 2 months, then retest hs-CRP.

4. **Green tea:** Recent research has found that the catechin antioxidants in green tea help to increase fat burning while also reducing the risk of cancer, high cholesterol and diabetes. Besides its natural anti-inflammatory effects, green tea may also lower blood

sugar by inhibiting enzymes that allow starch and fat absorption from the intestine. Green tea contains theanine, which has a calming yet energizing effect on the body. Typical dosage is 3 to 4 cups of green tea a day or a 300 to 400 mg capsule of green tea extract one to three times daily. Green tea is one of my favorite choices for supporting weight loss and cutting inflammation. It can also be an enjoyable alternative if you are trying to cut coffee consumption.

Level Two Treatment
Hormonal Imbalance 1: Excess Insulin

A high score for Hormone Imbalance 1 indicates excess insulin (or insulin resistance) is a factor that could be interfering with your weight-loss goals. Although insulin plays an essential role in healthy body function, an excess of it will certainly make you fat. Too much insulin not only encourages your body to store unused glucose as fat, but also blocks the use of stored fat as an energy source. For these reasons, an abnormally high insulin level makes losing fat, especially around the abdomen, next to impossible.

SUPPLEMENT OPTIONS:

1. **Metabolic Repair Pack—Insulin Balancing Formula (Clear Medicine)**: I got so tired of prescribing a slew of individual supplements to get insulin under control and rejuvenate the metabolism that I combined the best treatment solutions to make my own formula to support insulin metabolism. Take 1 dose with breakfast and lunch. It contains green tea, which is great for boosting energy and fat loss, but it can keep you awake if consumed too close to bedtime.

2. **Resveratrim—Extra Strength Resveratrol Complex (Clear Medicine)**: Now you have access to the many benefits of red wine—without the wine bottle. A number of studies show this natural red wine extract assists with weight loss. Have you heard of the French Paradox—the fact that the French seem to eat and drink what they

want but still remain slim? This may be due to the resveratrol from all that red wine! Now we have access to this in a bottle and it's not a wine bottle. Data published in *Nature* (November 2006) showed that resveratrol protected mice from the harmful effects of a high-calorie diet, including heart disease, weight gain and diabetes. Resveratrol appears to act on adiponectin and also possesses natural anti-inflammatory properties. Adiponectin is produced by our fat cells but actually helps lose fat by improving our insulin sensitivity. I developed Resveratrim, which is a bio flavonoid complex containing three synergistic antioxidants: pterostilbene (methylated resveratrol), resveratrol and quercetin. With five to eight times better absorption than other resveratrol products, the components in Resveratrim has benefits for cardiovascular health, insulin sensitivity, neurological health, anti-aging and anti-inflammation. Take 1 pill one to two times a day on an empty stomach or away from food.

3. **Clear CLA—Metabolic Enhancement Formula (Clear Medicine):** CLA is naturally present in dairy products and beef. It has anti-cancer and antidiabetic properties and may be useful in reducing arterial disease, as well as osteoporosis. "Dietary Fat Intake, Supplements and Weight Loss," published in the *Canadian Journal of Applied Physiology* (December 2000), reported that CLA is one of only a few supplements proven to reduce body fat and assist in increasing lean muscle mass without a change in caloric intake. These powerful effects are due to its insulin-sensitizing properties. CLA also shows anti-inflammatory benefits and seems to reduce fat storage in the fat cells while also increasing fat-burning activity in the skeletal muscle. The minimum dosage is 1,500 mg twice daily with food for at least 3 months. CLA is one of my favorite choices for the treatment of insulin resistance and inflammation. It's also my top choice for preserving precious muscle during weight loss.

4. **Holy basil:** This important herb has been found to reduce cortisol and help the body adapt to stress. It also improves blood

sugar balance and the activity of insulin in the body. Take 2 gel caps each day. Holy basil is my favorite choice for aiding insulin resistance when stress is also a factor.

5. **Cinnamon:** Besides adding a nice flavor to cooking and baking, cinnamon has wonderful insulin-balancing effects. A study published in *Diabetes Care* (December 2003) showed that cinnamon may cause muscle and liver cells to respond more readily to insulin. Add 1 to 2 g to your food or drinks each day.

6. **Alpha-lipoic acid:** This supplement improves our cellular response to insulin. It has favorable effects on blood sugar balance, abdominal fat, aging and all of the complications of metabolic syndrome. Take 200 mg one to three times daily, with or without food. Note that taking my Metabolic Repair Pack (Clear Medicine) will provide you with a high-dose of alpha lipoic acid, green tea, cinnamon and all of the minerals that aid insulin balance (listed below).

7. **Minerals**

   - **Chromium:** As a key mineral involved in regulating the body's response to insulin, chromium deficiency may result in insulin resistance. Chromium picolinate, the most absorbable form of chromium, may help weight loss because of its positive effect on insulin response. Dosage is typically 200 to 400 mcg per day. Prediabetics or patients with type 2 diabetes often benefit from 800 to 1,000 mcg per day.
   - **Magnesium:** Most insulin-resistant patients have a magnesium deficiency. Magnesium improves our cellular response to insulin, stabilizes blood sugar, prevents cravings and reduces anxiety. Take 200 to 400 mg of magnesium glycinate a day. To treat and prevent constipation, increase to 600 to 800 mg per day, to bowel tolerance.
   - **Biotin:** This mineral is involved in the action of insulin. Take 300 mcg to 3 g per day.

- **Zinc:** This is essential for blood sugar balance and insulin action. Take 25 to 50 mg a day with food.

Hormonal Imbalance 2: Low Dopamine

If you had a high score for Hormone Imbalance 2 on your Hormonal Health Profile, your dopamine could be drained. Dopamine is the neurotransmitter that's heavily involved in the pleasure center within the brain. It is released in high amounts during activities such as eating, sex and other naturally enjoyable experiences. Many researchers today agree that dopamine is one of the reasons that foods can be addictive. We also know stress stimulates the production of dopamine, which provides us with more energy, drive and motivation, just as the addictive stimulants chocolate, caffeine, sugar and cigarettes can.

SUPPLEMENT OPTIONS:

1. **Clear Energy—Dopamine Support Formula (Clear Medicine):** Revitalize your brain, energy and metabolism with this herbal combination that specifically provides a wonderful dose of dopamine. I blended L-tyrosine, D-phenylalanine and rhodiola to boost your metabolic power and brain energy. Take 2 to 3 pills on rising, before breakfast.

2. **L-Tyrosine:** The amino acid tyrosine is a building block of dopamine, so supplements can definitely help perk up production of this important mood-influencing hormone. Take 500 to 1,000 mg on rising, away from food. Another dose may be added later in the day, but because tyrosine is a stimulating supplement, it should not be taken after 3 p.m. and should be avoided completely by anyone with high blood pressure. This product should be taken for at least 4 to 6 weeks to reach full effectiveness. Tyrosine is the *best* choice if low thyroid hormone or underactive thyroid is also suspected.

3. **D- or DL-Phenylalanine:** Like tyrosine, phenylalanine is a building block of dopamine. A study published in one German psychiatry

journal showed that phenylalanine was as effective as certain anti-depressant drugs. Take 500 to 1,000 mg a day, away from food, before 3 p.m. As with tyrosine, phenylalanine must be taken for at least 4 to 6 weeks for full effectiveness. DL-phenylalanine may be the better choice if you also have body aches and pains.

4. **Rhodiola:** Rhodiola can enhance learning capacity and memory and may also be useful for treating fatigue, stress and depression. Research suggests rhodiola may enhance mood regulation and fight depression by stimulating the activity of serotonin and dopamine. Take 200 to 400 mg per day in the morning, away from food, for a minimum of 1 month.

5. **Chasteberry (Vitex):** Chasteberry has been shown to increase both dopamine and progesterone, making it an excellent choice for women who experience symptoms of depression in conjunction with PMS or irregular menstrual cycles. Take 200 mg of a 10:1 extract each morning before breakfast for 1 to 6 months.

FOODS AND SPECIFIC HABITS THAT INCREASE DOPAMINE:

- All proteins (meat, milk products, fish, beans, nuts, soy products). Turkey is high in phenylalanine. In fact, phenylalanine is found in most protein-rich foods, so eat them when you want to feel sharper. Coffee may also stimulate dopamine release, but remember to not go overboard on the caffeine!
- Exercise.
- Sex.
- Massage.
- Sources of tyrosine to increase the production of dopamine include almonds, avocados, bananas, dairy products, lima beans, pumpkin seeds and sesame seeds.

Hormonal Imbalance 3: Low Serotonin

Balancing serotonin is critical for effective weight loss. Though serotonin is typically recognized as a brain chemical, most of this neurotransmitter is produced in our digestive tract. Serotonin exerts a powerful influence over mood, emotions, memory, cravings (especially for carbohydrates!), self-esteem, pain tolerance, sleep habits, appetite, digestion and body temperature regulation. When we're depressed or down, we naturally crave more sugars and starches to stimulate the production of serotonin. By now, we all understand that excess carb consumption causes weight gain and possibly insulin resistance. While antidepressant medications such as selective serotonin re-uptake inhibitors (SSRIs) are effective in raising serotonin in the short term, some evidence suggests these medications actually deplete serotonin over time. Furthermore, weight gain is one of the most common side effects of antidepressant drugs.

SUPPLEMENT OPTIONS:

1. **Clear Mood—Serotonin Support Formula (Clear Medicine):** This effective formula contains all of the ingredients to increase your serotonin for better mood, appetite, sleep, digestion, memory and pain relief. I have included vitamin B6, 5-HTP and folic acid. Take 2 to 4 capsules before bed, and/or 1 or 2 capsules in the morning. If the capsules make you feel nauseated when taken on an empty stomach in the morning, try it with your protein smoothie or at bedtime instead.

2. **5-HTP:** A derivative of tryptophan and one step closer toward becoming serotonin, 5-HTP has been found to be more effective than tryptophan for treating sleeplessness, depression, anxiety and fibromyalgia. Take 50 to 400 mg a day, in divided doses throughout the day or before bed. This product should be taken for at least 4 to 6 weeks to reach full effectiveness.

3. **Vitamin B6:** Vitamin B6 supports the production and function of serotonin in the brain. Take 50 to 100 mg before bed.

4. **Rhodiola:** Rhodiola may enhance learning capacity, memory and mood regulation. It may also help fight depression by stimulating

the activity of serotonin and dopamine. Take 200 to 400 mg each day, preferably in the morning.

5. **St. John's Wort:** This herb has been proven effective for easing mild to moderate depression. It appears to work as a natural SSRI by preventing the breakdown of serotonin in the brain. It takes at least 4 to 6 weeks to reach full effectiveness. Recommended dosage is 900 mg a day, away from food.

6. **Inositol:** Naturally present in many foods, inositol improves the activity of serotonin in the brain. As a supplement, it is an excellent choice for alleviating anxiety and depression and supporting nervous system health. I use it in powdered form and add it to my daily smoothie. Take 4 to 12 g a day. When mixed with magnesium, inositol is very effective for calming the nervous system.

FOODS AND SPECIFIC HABITS THAT INCREASE SEROTONIN:

- Eating carbohydrates will boost your serotonin. Choose slow-release, complex carbs, including whole-grain breads, brown rice or pasta, to keep you sustained, energized and balanced. Simple carbs such as white bread and pastries will give you only a momentary boost followed by a crash. Plus they pack on the fat!
- The best food sources of serotonin-boosting tryptophan are brown rice, cottage cheese, meat, peanuts and sesame seeds.
- Chia seed contains tryptophan too.
- Meditating or focusing your mind on one thing. Avoid multitasking!
- Sun exposure (in moderation!).
- Staying warm.
- Exercise.
- Massage.

Hormonal Imbalance 4: Low GABA

Gamma-aminobutyric acid (GABA) is a naturally calming, inhibitory neurotransmitter involved in relaxation, healthy sleep, digestion and the easing of muscle tension, pain and anxiety. GABA appears to regulate the activity of stimulating the neurotransmitters dopamine, serotonin and noradrenaline. It calms us and indirectly helps with fat loss because of its beneficial effects on sleep, mood and reduction of stress and tension.

SUPPLEMENT OPTIONS:

1. **Clear Calm—GABA Enhancing Formula (Clear Medicine):** Inositol, GABA, taurine and passionflower help make this the perfect formula to ease tension, improve sleep and reduce anxiety. Take 2 to 3 capsules in the evening, before bed.

2. **GABA:** GABA is an inhibitory neurotransmitter, a brain chemical that has a calming effect. If you are anxious, have trouble sleeping and experience muscle tension or pain, this supplement is a good choice for you. Take 500 to 2,000 mg about an hour or two before bed. Alternatively, take GABA 10 to 20 minutes before meals, beginning with your evening meal. The standard dose of 200 mg three times daily can be increased to a maximum of 450 mg three times daily, if needed. This latter dosage should not be exceeded.

3. **Passionflower:** This calming herb appears to improve the activity of GABA. It is an excellent choice for anxiety and sleep disruption, even in children. Take 300 to 500 mg at bedtime.

4. **Taurine:** This amino acid plays a major role in the brain as an inhibitory neurotransmitter. Similar in structure and function to GABA, taurine provides a similar antianxiety effect that helps calm or stabilize an excited brain. Taurine is also effective for treating migraines, insomnia, agitation, restlessness, irritability, alcoholism, obsessions, depression and even hypomania/mania (the "high" phase of bipolar disorder or manic depression). Take 500 to 1,000 mg a day. Taking your last dose before bed is often most helpful. Taurine should be taken without food.

5. **Magnesium:** Our calming mineral, magnesium has wonderful

relaxing effects on our tense muscles, racing mind and overactive nervous system. Take 200 to 400 mg each day.

- Fish (especially mackerel) and wheat bran
- Relaxation
- Sleep
- Yoga
- Massage

Level Three Treatment
Hormonal Imbalance 5: Excess Cortisol

A high score for Hormone Imbalance 5 in your Hormonal Health Profile suggests stress is negatively affecting your metabolism and your health. Unlike adrenaline, which draws on your fat stores for energy during stressful situations, cortisol consumes your metabolically active muscle tissue for fuel. Prolonged stress can, therefore, lead to muscle wasting and high blood sugar simply because your body is struggling to adapt. When these conditions take over, stress becomes extremely destructive to your metabolism, body composition and wellness. Cortisol also depresses your metabolic rate by blocking your thyroid hormone, fuels your desire for fatty foods and carbohydrates and boosts abdominal fat storage.

SUPPLEMENT OPTIONS:

1. **Clear Balance—Stress Modifying Formula (Clear Medicine):** My favorite formula to beat stress and increase your energy. This powerful herbal combination also helps your body recuperate from chronic stress. Take 1 to 2 capsules once or twice daily, away from food.

2. **Vitamin C:** Vitamin C is naturally highest in our adrenal glands, and research suggests that just 20 minutes of stress can deplete our vitamin C stores! Vitamin C is a potent antioxidant, essential

for healthy immune system function and collagen formation in the skin, tendons and ligaments. Take 2,000 to 6,000 mg per day for stress protection and immune support. Ensure your vitamin C contains bioflavonoids, which enhance the activity of vitamin C in the body.

3. **B vitamins:** Endurance athletes and stressed or fatigued individuals should take extra B vitamins, especially pantothenic acid, which helps the body adapt to stress and supports adrenal gland function. When taken at bedtime, vitamin B6 is also useful in correcting abnormally high cortisol release throughout the night. B vitamins are water soluble and are easily depleted with perspiration and stress. Take 200 to 500 mg of vitamin B5 and/or 50 to 100 mg of B6 every day. These are often available in combination.

4. **Relora:** This supplement is a mixture of the herbal extracts *Magnolia officinalis* and *Phellodendron amurense*. It is medically proven to reduce stress and anxiety. It significantly reduces cortisol and raises DHEA, sometimes within as little as 2 weeks of use. Relora can be used to prevent health conditions associated with stress, including poor immunity, high blood pressure, insomnia or sleep disruption, loss of vitality and weight gain, especially in relation to metabolic syndrome. Take 2 capsules, 250 mg each, at bedtime and 1 capsule upon rising for at least a month. Relora is best taken away from food. I find the most effective formulas include a mixture of B vitamins and folic acid, like the Clear Balance—Stress Modifying Formula (Clear Medicine).

5. **Ashwagandha:** Ayurvedic practitioners use this herb to enhance mental and physical performance, improve learning ability and decrease stress and fatigue. Ashwagandha is a general tonic that can be used in stressful situations, especially insomnia, restlessness or when you are feeling overworked. The typical dosage is 500 to 1,000 mg twice a day for a minimum of 1 to 6 months. Capsules should be standardized to 1.5 percent with anolides per

dose. Ashwagandha is my favorite choice for reducing cortisol, increasing thyroid hormones and treating stress with a sluggish metabolism, anxiety, poor concentration and tension.

6. **Holy basil:** Holy basil has been found to reduce cortisol and help the body adapt to stress. It also improves blood sugar balance and the activity of insulin in the body. Holy basil is my favorite choice for reducing cortisol when insulin resistance or hypoglycemia symptoms are also present. Take 2 gel caps a day for at least a month.

7. **Hydrolyzed milk protein:** No matter whether the stress you are under is physical, emotional, psychological or environmental, milk protein hydrolysate is documented to prevent the associated rise in cortisol by calming the stress response pathway. Dosage is 75 to 300 mg a day. I love this supplement, and patients consistently report that it simply "takes the edge off."

8. **Phosphatidylserine (PS):** This supplement is ideal for alleviating nighttime worrying. It curbs the inappropriate release of stress hormones and protects the brain from the negative effects of cortisol, such as memory loss and poor concentration. PS may also reduce the negative effects of cortisol on muscle tissues during exercise. Take 100 to 200 mg before bed.

9. **Rhodiola:** This herbal supplement can enhance learning capacity and memory and may also be useful for treating fatigue, stress and depression. Research suggests rhodiola may enhance mood regulation and fight depression by stimulating the activity of serotonin and dopamine. Take 200 to 400 mg a day in the morning, away from food, for at least 6 weeks. Rhodiola is my favorite choice for reducing cortisol, increasing serotonin and dopamine and eliminating stress and anxiety, depression, cravings, fatigue and poor concentration, and even symptoms of ADHD. I personally take 3 capsules of Clear Energy (Clear Medicine) upon rising each morning for a good dose of rhodiola to help lower stress and improve mood and focus.

Hormonal Imbalance 6: Low Cortisol (Adrenal Gland Fatigue or Adrenal Gland Burnout)

Adrenal gland burnout is another consequence of constant stress. If you always feel tense or anxious, your body will remain in a constant state of heightened arousal. Constantly overproducing cortisol and adrenaline day after day because of ongoing stress, multitasking, skipping meals, excessive calorie restriction, insufficient carbohydrate intake, too much protein consumption, lack of sleep or too much coffee will lead to adrenal gland burnout. In this state, your adrenal glands simply can't keep up with the constant stimulation and outrageous demands for adrenaline and cortisol production, so they simply shut down. When your adrenal glands go on strike, cortisol and adrenaline levels plummet, resulting in chronic fatigue, lack of stamina for exercise, increased allergy symptoms, sleep disruption, blood sugar imbalances, depression, more cravings and weakened immunity.

SUPPLEMENT OPTIONS:
1. **Licorice extract:** Licorice Plus from Metagenics can help to raise cortisol levels. I normally prescribe 3 capsules upon rising, away from food.
2. **Isocort (Bezwecken):** This is a strong adrenal extract. Each capsule contains 2.5 mg of hydrocortisone, according to the manufacturer. Standard dosing is upon rising, noon and around 3 to 4 p.m. No more than 8 capsules a day should be used. I do not recommend the use of this product without salivary testing, which will clearly identify low cortisol. See your MD or ND.
3. **Cortrex (Thorne Research):** This supplement contains a mixture of licorice and adrenal gland extracts. It is very energizing. Take 1 to 2 capsules at breakfast and another at lunch.

FOODS AND SPECIFIC HABITS THAT INCREASE CORTISOL:
- Avoid excessive exercise, which will only exacerbate adrenal gland fatigue.

- Get adequate rest.
- Follow the Glyci-Med dietary approach.

Hormonal Imbalance 7: Low DHEA

Produced by the adrenal glands, DHEA is a precursor to the sex hormones estrogen and testosterone and is also one of the most abundant hormones in our body. It is known to support healthy immunity (particularly autoimmune function), aid tissue repair, improve sleep and counteract the negative effects of cortisol. It influences our ability to lose fat and gain muscle. It boosts libido and helps us feel motivated, youthful and energetic—just a few of the reasons that DHEA is often touted as the antiaging hormone.

SUPPLEMENT OPTIONS:

1. **Clear Balance—Stress Modifying Formula (Clear Medicine):** The main ingredient in this product, relora, significantly reduces cortisol and raises DHEA within only 2 weeks of use. Relora can be used to prevent the health conditions associated with stress, including poor immunity, high blood pressure, insomnia or sleep disruption, loss of vitality and weight gain, especially in relation to metabolic syndrome. Take 2 capsules, 250 mg each, 1 at bedtime and 1 on rising. It is best taken away from foods.

2. **DHEA:** You may purchase supplements of DHEA over the counter in the United States but its sale is restricted in Canada. DHEA should be taken under medical supervision by a licensed health-care provider. I prefer low dosages of 5 to 25 mg twice daily with meals. You should test your DHEA levels after 4 to 6 weeks of taking the supplement to avoid taking in excessive amounts, which can be harmful.

3. **7-Keto DHEA:** Unlike straight DHEA, 7-Keto DHEA does not convert to estrogen or testosterone, making it a good choice for younger people who, in most cases, would not benefit from increased amounts of these hormones. 7-Keto enhances

metabolism effects, promotes fat loss, protects us from the harmful effects of excess cortisol and appears to prevent the decrease in the metabolism known to occur when we're dieting. Take 25 to 100 mg twice a day. The higher dosage has been proven effective for weight loss in clinical trials, according to a report in *Current Therapeutic Research* (2000).

FOODS AND SPECIFIC HABITS THAT INCREASE DHEA:

- Meditation
- Exercise, specifically weight training
- Sex
- Sleep
- Managing stress

Level Four Treatment

Hormonal Imbalance 8: Excess Estrogen

Estrogen balance is essential for achieving and maintaining fat loss. In men and premenopausal women, estrogen dominance causes toxic fat gain, water retention, bloating and a host of other health and wellness issues. While premenopausal women with too much estrogen tend to have the pear-shape body type with more weight at the hips, both men and menopausal women with this excess exhibit an apple shape with more fat accumulation in the abdominal area. Researchers have now identified excess estrogen to be just as great a risk factor for obesity—in both sexes—as poor eating habits and lack of exercise.

SUPPLEMENT OPTIONS:

1. **Clear Detox—Hormonal Health and Clear Detox—Digestive Health (Clear Medicine).** Take 1 pack of Hormonal Health before breakfast and 1 pack of Digestive Health before bed each with a full glass of water. Be sure to use these products with a probiotic supplement such as Clear Flora to enhance the effectiveness of the detoxification process. The use of these two detox

packs provide all of the nutrients and herbs required for liver and toxic estrogen detoxification.

2. **Indole-3-carbinol (I3C):** Formulated from extracts of broccoli and other cruciferous vegetables, I3C is known to increase the breakdown and excretion of harmful estrogen metabolites. It may also be useful in the treatment and prevention of breast and prostate cancers. Take 200 mg twice a day for 1 to 3 months.

3. **Calcium D-glucarate:** This calcium salt is heavily involved in detoxification and the removal of estrogen from the body. Some evidence suggests it protects against cancers of the colon, breast and prostate. Take 500 mg twice a day for 1 to 3 months.

4. **Turmeric, rosemary extract, green tea and milk thistle:** Together these herbs support the elimination of estrogen by enhancing the liver detoxification pathways. Look for a product containing a mixture of all these ingredients, such as Clear Detox— Hormonal Health (Clear Medicine).

5. **Magnesium:** One of the many supporting ingredients in my detox formula, magnesium is helpful for detoxing excess estrogen and alleviating PMS. Ovarian hormones influence magnesium levels, triggering decreases at certain times during the menstrual cycle as well as altering the calcium-to-magnesium ratio. These cyclical changes can produce many of the well-known symptoms of PMS in women who are deficient in magnesium and/or calcium. For best results, take 200 to 600 mg a day throughout the month.

FOODS AND SPECIFIC HABITS THAT DECREASE HARMFUL ESTROGEN:

- Consume weak phytoestrogenic foods such as pomegranate, flaxseed, pears, apples, berries, organic non-GMO fermented soy, wheat germ, oats and barley.
- Eat yogurt and high-fiber foods to aid the breakdown and elimination of estrogen.
- Choose organic dairy and meat products to reduce your exposure to hormone additives.

- Add plenty of detoxifying foods to your diet, including broccoli, cauliflower, Brussels sprouts, kale, cabbage, beets, carrots, apples, ginger, onions and celery.
- Avoid alcohol.
- Avoid exposure to xenoestrogens from plastics, cosmetics and the birth control pill.
- Avoid unfermented soy products.
- Use infrared sauna treatments regularly to rid your body of toxins.
- Get plenty of exercise.
- Maintain a lower body-fat percentage (remember your fat produces harmful estrogen).

Hormonal Imbalance 9: Low Estrogen (Low Estrogen = More Belly Fat for Women)

While the effects of excess estrogen are clearly very real and detrimental, too little estrogen also has negative impacts on health and appearance. As estrogen levels drop off, especially during menopause, many women find themselves battling that oh-so-lovely shift in body fat from the hips to the waist. Since estrogen helps our cells respond better to insulin, a plunge in estrogen also tends to cause an unwelcome increase in insulin.

SUPPLEMENT OPTIONS:

1. **Bi-est bioidentical cream:** This topical cream is a mix of 80 percent estriol and 20 percent estradiol. See your MD, ND or compounding pharmacy. The dosage will depend on your specific condition. I recommend applying the cream to areas of thin skin (e.g., wrist, elbow crease, behind the knees, neck, etc.) rather than over fatty tissue where it may accumulate (e.g., inner thigh, abdomen, back of the arms).
2. **Phytoestrogenic herbs:** Black cohosh, angelica, red clover extract, sage or licorice can be used to support healthy estrogen balance.

Use one or more of these to help with the symptoms of menopause and low estrogen.

- **Black cohosh** can be used to treat hot flashes, night sweats, vaginal dryness, urinary urgency and other symptoms that can occur during menopause. Take 40 mg twice daily, away from food.
- **Angelica** has been used for many years to treat many symptoms of menopause (hot flashes, etc.), lack of menstrual cycle (amenorrhea) and PMS. It is anti-inflammatory and may help to relieve menstrual cramps due to its antispasmodic properties. Take 400 mg one to three times a day, away from food.
- **Red clover** contains high quantities of plant-based estrogens called isoflavones that may improve menopausal symptoms, reduce the risk of bone loss and lower the risk of heart disease by improving blood pressure and increasing HDL cholesterol. Research on the effectiveness of red clover for the treatment of menopause has yielded conflicting evidence—some reports show it is beneficial, while others claim it is no more helpful than a placebo. You can try taking 80 mg of red clover each day to see if it does the trick for you. Look for Promensil, which appears to be the most extensively researched product.
- **Sage** is an excellent choice to support healthy estrogen balance, especially if sweating and hot flashes are your predominant menopausal symptoms. Take 300 to 400 mg once a day, away from food.
- **Licorice** has phytoestrogenic properties and is an especially great choice if you're feeling burned out or stressed. Take 300 to 900 mg a day before 3 p.m. Because licorice is stimulating, it should not be taken later in the day and should be avoided completely if you have high blood pressure.
- **Clear Estrogen—Hormone Balancing Formula (Clear**

Medicine): Sometimes a blend of estrogenic herbs works best. This formula contains most of the herbs listed on the previous page. Take 2 capsules a day, but decrease the dosage if you experience breast pain or swelling.

FOODS AND SPECIFIC HABITS THAT IMPROVE THE SYMPTOMS OF LOW ESTROGEN:

- Phytoestrogenic foods such as soy products, flaxseed, fennel, pomegranate, etc.

Hormonal Imbalance 10: Low Progesterone

Progesterone is a natural diuretic, sleep aid, antianxiety compound and stimulator of metabolism (because it supports thyroid hormone). It's also considered to be thermogenic because it raises body temperature. Progesterone may help to build bone density, reduce blood pressure, lower LDL cholesterol, improve the appearance and texture of hair and skin, aid libido and prevent PMS.

SUPPLEMENT OPTIONS:

1. **Clear Progesterone—Hormone Balancing Formula (Clear Medicine):** This formula contains a combination of progesterone-supporting herbs and others that support optimal progesterone function. If you are a premenopausal woman, it can be taken during days 14 to 28 of your cycle for PMS symptoms or throughout the whole menstrual cycle, if needed. Normal dose is 1 to 3 capsules a day, away from food, preferably upon rising.

2. **Bioidentical progesterone cream:** I prefer a 3 to 6 percent natural progesterone cream. See your MD, ND or compounding pharmacy. If you are using this product for PMS, apply it on days 14 to 28 of your cycle, when progesterone is naturally highest. For the treatment of menopause symptoms, it may be used for 25 days followed by 5 days off, or it may be applied on a schedule that more closely matches a woman's natural menstrual cycle. I recommend

applying the cream to areas of thin skin (e.g., wrist, elbow crease, behind the knees, neck, etc.) rather than over fatty tissue where it may accumulate (e.g., inner thigh, abdomen, back of the arms).

3. **Chasteberry extract (Vitex):** Chasteberry increases progesterone by stimulating the production of lutenizing hormone. Take 200 mg per day, away from food, for 1 to 6 months.

4. **Evening primrose oil:** While flaxseed oil appears to be estrogen enhancing, EPO is touted as a progesterone-enhancing compound. Take 1,000 to 2,000 mg a day.

Hormonal Imbalance 11: Excess Progesterone

Progesterone excess is rare, though I often see it in individuals who use progesterone creams or pills. Too much progesterone can cause acne, bloating, water retention, depression and weight gain.

SUPPLEMENT OPTIONS:

1. **Clear Detox—Hormonal Health and Clear Detox—Digestive Health (Clear Medicine)**, listed above for high estrogen, also can be helpful for excess progesterone.

2. **Hydrolyzed milk protein:** Progesterone may also rise when the stress response is chronically overstimulated. Supplements of hydrolyzed milk protein, which decreases stimulation of the stress response pathway, may indirectly help to reduce excess progesterone.

3. **Avoid evening primrose oil,** since it appears to increase progesterone.

Hormonal Imbalance 12: Low Testosterone

Loss of testosterone with aging can lead to andropause, often referred to as male menopause. This condition is estimated to affect about 30 percent of aging men, although actual numbers may be much higher because the widely varying symptoms make definitive diagnosis difficult. The symptoms of testosterone imbalance illustrate how testosterone decline tends to cause an increase in body fat and loss of muscle. I should add that these effects can arise both in men *and* women, even with dieting and exercise, when a marked deficiency of testosterone exists.

SUPPLEMENT OPTIONS:

1. **Clear Testosterone—Hormone Balancing Formula (Clear Medicine):** Clear Testosterone contains a blend of herbs to support the body during stress (a major killer of testosterone!) and other herbs designed to help promote optimal testosterone production and function. Take 1 to 2 per day upon rising, away from food.

2. **Bioidentical testosterone cream:** See your MD, ND or compounding pharmacy.

3. **Clear Detox—Hormonal Health (Clear Medicine):** Because excess estrogen is often associated with a deficiency of testosterone in men, my detox formulation can be helpful, since it helps with the removal of harmful estrogen.

4. *Tribulus terrestris*: Also known as puncture vine, *Tribulus* may boost testosterone by increasing the secretion of lutenizing hormone (LH) from the pituitary gland. Other studies suggest it boosts testosterone by increasing DHEA. Take 500 to 1,000 mg a day, away from food.

5. **Arginine:** Arginine may improve testosterone. Take 3,000 mg a day, away from food, preferably at bedtime.

6. **Zinc:** This mineral is needed to maintain testosterone levels in the blood. A deficiency of zinc causes a decrease in the activity of LH, the hormone that stimulates the production of testosterone. Zinc also appears to inhibit the conversion of testosterone to estrogen via the aromatase enzyme. Take 25 to 50 mg a day with food.

FOODS AND SPECIFIC HABITS THAT INCREASE TESTOSTERONE:

- Sleep
- Exercise

- Sex
- Exposure to morning sunlight
- Protein
- Sufficient fat and avoidance of excess carbohydrate restriction
- Cuddling (women)
- Competitive sports (men)
- Winning a business deal, success in competitive activities or ventures

Hormonal Imbalance 13: Excess Testosterone

While excess testosterone is not very common in men, it affects about 10 percent of women. A surplus of female testosterone is typically a result of increased production by the adrenal glands and is associated with polycystic ovary syndrome (PCOS) and hirsutism (excess hair growth). Besides causing acne, facial hair growth and even male-pattern hair loss in women, too much testosterone increases insulin resistance and weight gain, causing the apple body type.

SUPPLEMENT OPTIONS:

1. **Saw palmetto:** This herb appears to inhibit the enzyme that supports the conversion of testosterone to dihydrotestosterone (DHT). It may also reduce the risk of prostate enlargement and hair loss commonly associated with DHT. Saw palmetto may boost a woman's breast size if shrinkage has occurred due to excess testosterone exposure. Take 160 mg twice a day. I have found great success treating acne and hair loss in women due to high testosterone with a formula called SP Ultimate (Pure Encapsulations). It contains saw palmetto as well as additional ingredients to aid testosterone balance.

2. **Options for Hormone Imbalances 1 and 5:** Because high testosterone in women is usually a result of excess insulin or cortisol, choose supplements that improve insulin sensitivity (Hormone

Imbalance 1) and lower cortisol (Hormone Imbalance 5) to restore testosterone balance.

3. **Options for liver detox and digestive detox, particularly Clear Detox—Hormonal Health and Clear Detox—Digestive Health (Clear Medicine):** Support of liver detoxification is also beneficial to aid the breakdown and elimination of testosterone. Therefore, milk thistle, calcium D-glucarate and turmeric can be helpful for this imbalance.

Level Five Treatment
Hormonal Imbalance 14: Low Thyroid Hormone

Thyroid hormones regulate our metabolism and organ function and directly affect heart rate, cholesterol levels, body weight, energy, muscle contraction and relaxation, skin and hair texture, bowel function, fertility, menstrual regularity, memory, mood and other body processes.

SUPPLEMENT OPTIONS:

1. **Clear Metabolism—Thyroid Support Formula (Clear Medicine):** Wake up your metabolism with this fantastic formula that supports thyroid hormone production and activity. I have combined the best thyroid-supporting ingredients, including iodine, potassium, L-tyrosine and ashwagandha. Take 2 to 3 capsules on rising, before breakfast.

2. **Ashwagandha:** This supplement may increase both thyroxine (T4) and its more potent counterpart, T3. Both ashwagandha and gugulipids appear to boost thyroid function without influencing the release of the pituitary hormone TSH (thyroid-stimulating hormone), indicating that these herbs work directly on the thyroid gland and other body tissues. Good news, since thyroid problems most often occur within the thyroid gland itself or in the conversion of T4 into T3 in tissues outside the thyroid gland. Take 750 to 1,000 mg twice a day. Ashwagandha is my favorite choice for supporting the thyroid when stress is also a concern.

3. **Forskohlin:** Extracted from the herb *Coleus forskohlii,* forskohlin may increase the release of thyroid hormone by stimulating substance cAMP. cAMP is comparable in strength to TSH, which prompts the thyroid to produce more hormone. Take 250 mg two to three times a day. Forskohlin is one of the top supplement choices when both weight loss and thyroid support are the goals.

4. **Gugulipids (*Commiphora mukul*):** Gugulipids enhance the conversion of T4 to the more potent form, T3. Dosage is 500 mg three times a day. Gugulipids may also lower elevated cholesterol and aid weight loss, so choose this one if you are concerned about high cholesterol or weight loss in addition to sluggish thyroid function.

5. **L-Tyrosine:** The amino acid tyrosine is necessary for the production of thyroid hormone in the body. Recommended dose is 1,000 mg on rising, before breakfast. *Do not take this supplement if you have high blood pressure.* My preference, should you wish to take L-tyrosine for thyroid health, is for you to consider using Clear Energy (Clear Medicine) (3 capsules on rising) because it also contains rhodiola. This indirectly helps with thyroid function because it lowers cortisol, which is known to suppress thyroid hormone activity.

FOODS AND SPECIFIC HABITS THAT INCREASE THYROID HORMONE:

- Exercise—but do not overexercise!
- Get plenty of sleep. Sleep deprivation decreases thyroid hormone and your metabolic rate.
- Eat regularly and avoid excessive caloric restriction.
- Consume foods that contain the nutrients necessary for the production of thyroid hormone:
  - Tyrosine—almonds, avocados, bananas, dairy products, pumpkin seeds and sesame seeds.
  - Iodine—fish (cod, sea bass and haddock), shellfish and sea vegetables such as seaweed and kelp. Kelp is the richest source of iodine.

- Selenium—brewer's yeast, wheat germ, whole grains (barley, whole wheat, oats and brown rice), seeds, nuts (especially Brazil nuts), shellfish and some vegetables (garlic, onions, mushrooms, broccoli, tomatoes and radishes).

Level Six Treatment
Hormonal Imbalance 15: Low Acetylcholine
Keeping acetylcholine levels high is one of the secrets to maintaining strong, healthy, metabolically active muscle. Acetylcholine also stimulates growth hormone release, thereby improving tissue healing, promoting muscle growth, improving skin tone and bone density and aiding fat loss (especially abdominal fat).

SUPPLEMENT OPTIONS:

1. **Acetyl-L-carnitine:** Acetyl-L-carnitine is a potent antioxidant for the brain. It is an anti-inflammatory that provides a source of the acetyl group needed to make acetylcholine, as well as L-carnitine, which assists with fat burning. Take 500 to 1,000 mg a day, preferably in the morning before breakfast. Acetyl-L-carnitine is my favorite choice for boosting acetylcholine, aiding weight loss and slowing aging of the brain

2. **Phosphatidylcholine (PC):** PC provides choline, which is needed to make acetylcholine. Take 1,200 to 2,400 mg a day with food. PC is my favorite choice for use during pregnancy. It supports development of the baby's brain and nervous system, and I swear the babies I see in my practice are smarter for it!

3. **DMAE:** DMAE (dimethylaminoethanol) is anti-inflammatory and antioxidant and increases the production of acetylcholine. It is useful for both cognitive function and for improving muscle contractions. Take 100 to 300 mg daily with food. As an aside, DMAE may also be used topically to improve skin tone and firmness.

4. **L-Alpha-glycerophosphocholine (alpha-GPC):** Glycerophosphocholine plays an important role in the synthesis of acetylcholine. It maintains neurological health and may also help to enhance

growth hormone. The standard dose is one to two 500 mg capsules a day, away from food.

- Exercise.
- Healthy fats and sources of choline such as lecithin, egg yolks, wheat germ, soybeans, organ meats (liver, kidney, etc.) and whole-wheat products.

Hormonal Imbalance 16: Low Melatonin

Melatonin is a powerful antioxidant that maintains youthfulness, improves sleep, perks up libido and boosts energy and resistance to infections. It affects your ability to fall asleep, stay asleep and your sleep quality. It also indirectly influences your body composition through its relationship with growth hormone.

SUPPLEMENT OPTIONS:
1. **Melatonin:** Take 0.5 to 3 mg under your tongue per day at bedtime to aid sleep.

FOODS AND SPECIFIC HABITS THAT INCREASE MELATONIN:
- Sleep in total darkness.
- Expose yourself to bright light immediately upon rising and during the day; keep the lights dim after dinner.
- Consume protein, particularly sources that contain the tryptophan needed to make melatonin, such as pumpkin seeds, chia seeds and walnuts.
- Follow the habits for healthy sleep outlined in *The Hormone Diet*.

Level Seven Treatment

Hormonal Imbalance 17: Low Growth Hormone

Growth hormone affects just about every cell in the body. Not surprisingly, it also has a major effect on our feelings, actions and appearance. Because this regenerative hormone tends to decline with age, growth hormone supplements are often promoted as a way to slow the effects of aging. Growth hormone is released during deep sleep and while we exercise. It's essential for tissue repair, muscle building, bone density and healthy body composition. A study from the *Journal of Clinical Endocrinology & Metabolism* (April 2007) linked abdominal obesity in postmenopausal women with low growth hormone secretion, elevated inflammatory markers and increased risk of cardiovascular disease.

SUPPLEMENT OPTIONS:

1. **Clear Recovery—Strength and Exercise Formula (Clear Medicine):** Out of all of my formulations, I think this just might be my favorite. Complete with three types of glutamine, creatine, branched-chain amino acids (BCAAs), resveratrol, berry extracts, minerals and loads of antioxidants, it aids recovery after exercise and the production of growth hormone. Take 1 serving in water after exercise or in the midafternoon if you need an energy boost. If you are extremely athletic, you can take 2 servings during or after weight-training sessions or endurance exercise.

2. **Specific amino acids:** The amino acid precursors to growth hormone are arginine, lysine, ornithine and glutamine. Supplements of these amino acids taken together before bed or after exercise may be useful to support growth hormone production. Aim for the following dosages:
   - L-Arginine: 2,000–3,000 mg per day
   - L-Glutamine: 2,000 mg per day
   - L-Ornithine: 2,000–6,000 mg per day
   - L-Lysine: 1,200 mg per day
   - L-Glycine: 1,000 mg per day
   - L-Tyrosine: 1,000 mg per day
   - These amino acids are most effective when combined with niacin, vitamin B6, vitamin C, calcium, zinc and potassium

- Sleep
- Exercise
- Consume sufficient protein
- Manage stress

HORMONE DIET SUCCESS STORY: JOANNE

"Reading *The Hormone Diet* was a very enlightening experience for me. Over the years I have touched on a number of various diet suggestions, but doing this program has taught me so much more. In particular, I learned how to eat for hormonal balance and end the confusion of what to buy when shopping. I'm feeling so much better and have more energy. I plan to continue the program with determination to reach my weight goal! I can't believe that in 4 short weeks I lost 20 pounds and gained 3 pounds of muscle. I lost 3 inches off my waist and hips. All the other measurements were greatly improved—even my blood pressure. In a month I have completely turned my health around!"

JOANNE

STATS	APR	MAY	LOST
Weight	216	198	18
Fat Mass	79.5	58.4	21.1
Body Fat	36%	29%	7%
BP	135/83	106/81	↓
Waist (inches)	42	39	3
Hips (inches)	44	41	3

INITIAL CHIEF COMPLAINTS:

1. Weight
2. Skin
3. Energy level
4. Overall health

RECOMMENDED HEALTH TESTS: WORKING WITH YOUR DOCTOR TO COMPLETE THE 30-DAY *SUPERCHARGED* HORMONE DIET PROGRAM

Health is not simply the absence of sickness.

HANNAH GREEN

Gaining a full sense of your hormonal status often requires benchmarking tests that can be performed by your health-care provider. Understanding the medical tests you should ask for definitely puts you in the driver's seat when it comes to managing your own wellness. I decided to include this information because we receive requests weekly via phone and email for the list of blood tests I recommend patients have completed by their doctor.

This chapter begins with a brief explanation of all of blood tests that I believe are helpful to incorporate into your yearly medical checkup. You will find the actual list of tests, which can be photocopied to take to your doctor, at the end of this chapter. This panel of blood tests is similar to those we complete for patients enrolled in our hormonal health program at Clear Medicine. It's very thorough!

Whether you request these tests at your annual checkup or when you are going through a particularly symptomatic period, I recommend asking for a *copy of your blood test results and keeping them in a folder.* It's helpful for you to compare your results yearly, since the goal is to make sure your values remain in the *optimal* range, and not just within *normal* range. Remember, significant changes can occur in your blood work from one year to the next, even without the appearance of obvious physical signs.

Tests for General Health, Immunity and Wellness

- **CBC.** Otherwise known as complete blood count, this is the totality of your red and white blood cells. It is optimal to have all of the values in the normal range. A low red blood cell count indicates anemia, often related to low iron, vitamin B12 or folic acid. A low white blood cell count can signal weakened immunity. Though these conditions are usually not serious, consulting with an ND may be a good idea to help you address imbalances in this category of blood tests. Our means of interpretation are often broader.
- **Liver function tests for AST, ALT and bilirubin.** These tests are used to identify liver disease and function. Your liver is vital for fat loss and wellness, as you've already discovered. Poor or sluggish liver function can interfere with fat loss, cause hormonal imbalance and increase your risk of disease. Normal values are within the reference range, but lower is better. Milk thistle, dandelion root, turmeric and artichoke are wonderful herbs for supporting the natural processes of the liver. If your levels are abnormal, take one or more of these herbs for 3 months, and then retest your enzymes to see if levels have improved.
- **Zinc.** Zinc is a cofactor involved in at least 70 different enzymatic reactions in the body. As an essential mineral involved in healthy immunity, blood sugar balance, thyroid function, collagen production, bone density, tissue healing and repair, antioxidant protection, prostate function and growth hormone and testosterone production, zinc is vital to good health. Zinc depletion is common with use of the birth control pill, corticosteroids and diuretics. Its absorption is greatly compromised when your stomach acid (HCl) levels

are low. Zinc deficiency causes decreased senses of taste and smell, poor wound healing, white spots on the fingernails, night blindness, low sperm count, hair loss, behavior or sleep problems, mental sluggishness, impaired immune function and dermatitis. Optimally, your levels should be toward the high end of the laboratory reference range. You may add a supplement of zinc citrate if your zinc is low. Purchase zinc citrate or a chelated form of zinc for optimal absorption, and be sure to take it with food to avoid nausea.

- **Copper.** Excess vitamin C and zinc can interfere with copper availability. A deficiency of copper may result in anemia (indistinguishable from iron deficiency); impaired formation of collagen, elastin and connective tissue proteins; osteoporosis and arterial wall defects. If you have cardiovascular disease, I recommend that you monitor your copper levels closely. While deficiencies are harmful, especially for cardiovascular health, it's often more common to have excess copper mainly due to medication use or supplements, or from copper leaching into drinking water from pipes. Symptoms of copper toxicity include depression, acne and hair loss. If you find your copper is low, your multivitamin should provide all that you need. If your copper is too high, take 30 to 50 mg of zinc daily to encourage its depletion.

Tests for Glycemic Control, Fat Loss, Diabetes and Heart Disease Risk

- **Fasting glucose and insulin.** Glucose and insulin are implicated in many age-related diseases, such as type 2 diabetes, hypoglycemia, carbohydrate metabolism, hypertension, heart disease, insulin resistance and stroke. These tests require a fasting blood level, which means a 10- to 12-hour fast is required before the collection of your blood sample. The optimal value for fasting blood glucose is less than 86 mg/dL.

A value of less than 5 mU/mL is optimal for fasting insulin. Insulin resistance is associated with a glucose reading greater than 100 mg/dL and fasting insulin greater than 5.

- **Two-hour post-prandial glucose and insulin.** During testing day at my clinic, all of our patients arrive fasting and complete their first blood draw. As soon as the blood is drawn, we feed them waffles, maple syrup and orange juice and have them wait for 2 hours before drawing another sample of blood. The first sign of insulin resistance is elevated insulin *after* a meal *followed by high fasting insulin*. Insulin tends to be abnormal *long before* blood sugars start to rise, typical of the diabetic state. Insulin resistance may be apparent with 2-hour glucose readings of more than 140 mg/dL and insulin levels of more than 30 mU/mL. If either your fasting or 2-hour test is abnormal, you need to focus on improving your body's sensitivity to insulin with nutrition, stress management, supplements and strength training. If you add the insulin-sensitizing supplements outlined on pages 184–86 to your regimen after the detox, you will meet all of these treatment requirements. Continue with the treatment program for 3 to 6 months, and then repeat the test.
- **Fasting triglycerides.** Triglycerides are a particular type of fat that is present in our bloodstream and arises from fats or carbohydrates taken in. Calories we ingest that are not used immediately by our tissues are converted to triglycerides and transported to our fat cells to be stored. Then your hormones regulate the release of triglycerides from fat stores to help meet the body's needs for energy between meals. Levels greater than 100 mg/dL are associated with insulin resistance.
- **Fasting cholesterol (total, HDL and LDL).** An optimal level of "good" cholesterol (HDL) should be between 55 and 150 mg/dL. "Bad" cholesterol (LDL) should be between 80 and 120 mg/dL to be safe, and total cholesterol should be less than 150 mg/dL. If

your cholesterol is too high, I recommend Metabolic Repair Pack (Clear Medicine) twice daily with meals along with red rice yeast extract, which has an effect much like the statin medications, without side effects.

- **Uric acid.** Normal levels are less than 5.0 mg/dL. High levels of uric acid cause gout, are linked to increased heart disease risk and are also a sign of insulin resistance.

- **HbA1c levels.** This is an indicator of blood sugar control over the previous 120 days. Ideal levels are less than 5.0. If the number is higher, it indicates your blood sugar control over the previous months has been less than optimal. Again, this is another marker of insulin resistance or poor glucose control.

- **Fasting homocysteine (optimal value: less than 6.3).** It's useful to test vitamin B12 (optimal value: more than 600) and folic acid (optimal value: more than 1,000) at the same time, since these substances are involved in the process of metabolism necessary to reduce homocysteine levels along with vitamin B6 and a compound called trimethylglycine. Homocysteine is an inflammatory protein that, if elevated in the blood, is a proven independent risk factor for heart disease, osteoporosis, Alzheimer's disease and stroke. Homocysteine has been found to increase with insulin resistance. Vitamin B12, found only in animal-source foods, is necessary for the formation and regeneration of red blood cells. It also promotes growth, increases energy, improves sleep and cognition and helps maintain a healthy nervous system. Folic acid helps protect against genetic damage and birth defects. It is needed for the utilization of sugar and amino acids, prevents some types of cancer, promotes healthier skin and helps protect against intestinal parasites and food poisoning. If your homocysteine is too high, include a complex of vitamin B6, vitamin B12 and folic acid in your daily vitamin regimen until your next physical exam.

- **Highly sensitive C-reactive protein.** Hs-CRP is a marker of inflammation and a risk factor for arterial disease. Levels tend to increase as body fat increases and with insulin resistance. An optimal value is less than 0.8, although the Life Extension Foundation recommends less than 0.55 mg/L for men and less than 1.5 mg/L for women. This test is also important for breast cancer survivors and should be tested along with fasting and 2-hour PC insulin levels. High CRP or insulin is associated with increased risk of recurrence.

- **Ferritin.** Abnormally high levels of the storage form of iron called ferritin can increase the risk of heart and liver disease in both men and women. They also appear to increase inflammation. Optimal levels should be close to 70 in women and 100 in men. Low levels of iron are associated with fatigue, hypothyroidism, decreased athletic performance, ADD/ADHD, restless leg syndrome and hair loss. If your ferritin is too high, you should speak to your doctor about the possibility of donating blood to help to reduce your levels into a more optimal range. If ferritin is too low, use a supplement of iron citrate with 1,000 mg of vitamin C. The citrate form of iron will not cause constipation.

Hormonal Assessments

Your hormones are best tested in the morning. If you are menstruating, you should have your blood drawn on day 3 of your cycle to get the best picture of your estrogen and ovarian reserve and on day 20 to 22 to investigate progesterone (day 1 = first day of bleeding). If you are male or menopausal, you can have your blood tests completed on any day.

Note that you can also assess your hormones via saliva hormone analysis. This is argued to be the more accurate way to measure hormones because it looks at the free component of hormones rather than those bound to carrier proteins. The free component of hormones is biologically active. I use both saliva and blood testing in my clinical practice. I will complete a patient's blood tests at least once a year and saliva once a year as well, especially once the patient begins treatment with bioidentical hormones. Monitoring blood levels can only decrease the risk of overdose.

- **Follicle-stimulating Hormone (FSH) and Lutenizing Hormone (LH).** These hormones are released from the pituitary gland and stimulate the ovaries and testes. High levels are found in menopause, infertility or amenorrhea, premature ovarian failure or testicular failure. Low levels indicate pituitary dysfunction. If your FSH or LH is elevated, you will need to replenish estrogen, progesterone and/or testosterone. An excess of LH relative to FSH is common with polycystic ovary syndrome (PCOS).

- **DHEAs.** DHEA is a precursor hormone to estrogen and testosterone. This adrenal hormone protects against the harmful effects of the stress hormone cortisol, is cardio-protective and crucial for healthy body composition. It tends to naturally decrease as we age. Most antiaging programs recommend the use of DHEAs; however, it should not be taken unless a true deficiency has been diagnosed via blood work. Follow-up testing should be completed to ensure there is no excess present after treatment. In some cases of PCOS, DHEA may be abnormally high, contributing to hair loss and male-pattern balding. Optimal levels should be above 225 mcg/dL or, more specifically, 300 to 400 mcg/dL for men and 225 to 350 mcg/dL for women.

- **Cortisol.** High levels (more than 15 mcg/dL) of cortisol are detrimental for almost every tissue and organ in the body. They cause destruction of muscle; increase calcium loss from bone; accelerate the process of aging and are linked to memory loss, anxiety, depression and low libido, along with an increase in the deposition of fat around the abdomen. Low levels (less than 9 mcg/dL) indicate adrenal gland burnout.

- **Free and total testosterone.** Many men with insulin resistance, obesity or sleep apnea have low levels of testosterone, which is known to increase the risk of heart disease. This deficiency also influences erectile function, libido, sense of well-being, mood and motivation. Maintaining testosterone levels is crucial for building muscle and losing fat. Optimal levels of free testosterone levels for men should be in the range of 7.2 to 24 mcg/dL; total testosterone 241 to 827 mcg/dL. In women, low testosterone is damaging to bone density, a healthy libido and aspects of memory (especially task-oriented memory). If testosterone is too high (often associated with PCOS or insulin resistance), hair loss, acne, increased risk of breast cancer or infertility may occur.

- **Estradiol and estrone.** Estrogen values will vary in women depending on age and point in the menstrual cycle. The optimal value for estrogen is 180 to 200 pg/mL for premenopausal women and 60 to 120 pg/mL for women in their late 40s and older. Men's estradiol should be less than 40 pg/mL. In both sexes, high estrogen encourages fat storage. Elevated levels of estrogen in men are typically found in cases of increased abdominal obesity because the fat cells here encourage the conversion of testosterone to estrogen. High levels of estrogen and low levels of testosterone set the stage for sexual dysfunction and prostate conditions and promote weight gain in men. In women, excess estrogen is associated with PMS, weight gain around the hips, uterine fibroids and other gynecological conditions, as well as increased risk of certain types of cancers. Estrogen is naturally highest in the first half of the menstrual cycle, before menopause. After menopause, levels are normally consistent and much lower. As estrogen levels decline, more abdominal weight gain can arise, since estrogen affects insulin sensitivity. Lower levels of estrogen are also associated with a decrease in serotonin, which can lead to depression, anxiety, worrying and sleep disruption. Low estrogen can cause hot flashes, night sweats, urinary urgency and frequency, insomnia, depression, failing memory (especially when attempting to think of a word or name), hair texture and skin elasticity changes, a thickening waistline, vaginal dryness and a low libido. Low estrogen also increases the risk of heart disease, diabetes, Alzheimer's disease and osteoporosis.

- **Progesterone.** Progesterone is naturally highest in the second half of the menstrual cycle, and normal values can range widely. Progesterone is protective against anxiety, PMS, fibrocystic breast disease and water retention. It also encourages fat burning and is crucial for fertility. Progesterone protects the prostate gland in men and may help to restore low DHEA levels. Decreased levels are associated with infertility, amenorrhea (lack of menstruation), fetal death and toxemia in pregnancy.
- **TSH, Free T3, Free T4 and thyroid antibodies.** These four tests are required to accurately assess the function of the thyroid gland, our master gland of metabolism. TSH should be less than 2.0 to be optimal, not the currently accepted 4.7 reported by most labs. T3 and T4 should be in the middle of your lab's reference range. Thyroid antithyroglobulin antibodies should be negative. Quite often I find elevated antibodies prior to abnormalities in TSH, T3 or T4, which may be an early signal of the development of thyroid disease. It's almost impossible to have low body fat along with an improperly diagnosed or managed case of hypothyroidism. Currently, it's estimated that 1 in 13 people suffer from hypothyroidism (underactive thyroid), with the majority of cases being missed because of

improper testing or interpretation of the blood results. There is an increase in the risk of obesity, heart disease and blood sugar abnormalities in hypothyroid cases. Often, hypothyroid patients also have high levels of homocysteine and cholesterol. If you are attempting to conceive, thyroid antibody abnormalities must be corrected to improve your chances of conception.

- **25-Hydroxy vitamin D3.** Vitamin D has proven immune-enhancing, cancer-protective, bone-building and insulin-regulating benefits. It is also important during pregnancy. Your levels should be over 125. If your vitamin D is low, add 2,000 to 5,000 IU of vitamin D3 each day to your regimen, in addition to your multivitamin and calcium/magnesium supplement.

- **IGF-1.** This is a marker of growth hormone status. Because it remains constant in the blood longer than HGH (which tends to fluctuate in response to various stimuli), it is a more accurate indicator of HGH deficiency and is also more precise for monitoring HGH therapy than testing HGH directly. An optimal IGF-1 value will range between 200 and 300 ng/mL. Growth hormone is essential to maintaining healthy bones, skin and hair, as well as strong, lean muscle mass. It tends to naturally decrease as we age; however, conditions such as sleep deprivation, diabetes, hypothyroidism, anorexia, insulin resistance and some cases of osteoporosis can cause levels to decline more rapidly.

In summary, the complete list of tests you can request from your doctor includes:

FOR GENERAL HEALTH, ENERGY AND METABOLISM:
25-OH vitamin D
AST, ALT, GGT
CBC

Copper

DHEAs, cortisol

Electrolytes

Ferritin

Folate

Free and total testosterone

IGF-1

TSH, free T3, free T4, thyroid antibodies

Uric acid

Vitamin B12

Zinc

FOR HEART HEALTH, STROKE RISK AND DIABETES RISK ASSESSMENT:

Fasting:

Glucose

Triglycerides

Insulin

Cholesterol panel (HDL, LDL, total)

hs-CRP

Homocysteine

HbA1c

FOR HORMONAL HEALTH ASSESSMENT FOR MENOPAUSAL WOMEN
AND MEN:

(Can be tested at any time)

FSH

LH

Estradiol

Progesterone

FOR HORMONAL HEALTH ASSESSMENT FOR PREMENOPAUSAL WOMEN:

(Tests should be completed on day 3 and/or 20 to 22 of your cycle.
Day 1 is your first day of bleeding. Day 3 assesses ovarian reserve and

estrogen levels, while day 20 assesses progesterone levels. Both are important for fertility and prevention of PMS.)

Estradiol

Progesterone

LH

FSH

Here are your instructions for the blood tests once you have received the requisition for the tests:

Go to the lab after fasting for 10 to 12 hours. Premenopausal women should go to the lab on the appropriate day of their cycle. Aim to be at the lab before 9 a.m. or 10 a.m. since your hormones fluctuate as the day goes on. If you are doing a post-prandial glucose test, then you will then return to the lab 2 hours later for a second blood draw after consuming a high-carb meal (e.g., pancakes/waffles, syrup and orange juice). During this 2-hour waiting period, do not consume additional food or exercise.

Once all your blood tests are completed, be sure to ask for a copy of all your results to keep for your records. That way, you and your caregiver can keep a close eye on changes in your values from one year to the next.

You've reached the end of Part One. I hope you implement my suggestions and use the support tools in Parts Two and Three to keep you balanced for a lifetime.

PART TWO

*Every day do something that
will inch you closer to a better tomorrow.*

DOUG FIREBAUGH

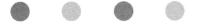

THE *SUPERCHARGED* HORMONE DIET—

WEEKLY MEAL PLANS AND PERMITTED FOOD LISTS

Your suggested meal plan for the coming 14-day detox, transition phase (food reintroduction) and final week of the Glyci-Med approach are presented in this section. During any given week, you are free to substitute any meal for another, but be sure to stick to the permitted foods for the week. Do *not* skip meals and be sure to consume an afternoon meal or shake daily. Pick and choose from any of the meal suggestions on any day, but take note of days designated for the reintroduction of specific foods during week 3. Note, also, the times at which you should aim to have all your meals and snacks.

I have tried not to repeat meals on consecutive days, but you will notice that most of the soups, snacks and dinner dishes provide more than 1 serving, so you can certainly spend a bit of time cooking for one day and enjoy tasty food for the following three. If you like, freeze the soups and chili in individual servings, so you have easy (and optional mid-morning) meals ready to go.

Your recommended mid-morning and mid-afternoon snack is a shake. If you prefer, you can choose to have the shake for breakfast and a mid-afternoon snack. In this case, just be sure to replace the mid-morning shake with a high-protein snack containing the foods you are allowed to have during each particular week (such as a hard-boiled egg with 5 to 6 almonds and cucumber slices).

Your Hormonal Health Detox Shake Options

For those of you who are 125 pounds or less, I recommend taking one detox shake per day in the afternoon. If your current weight is above this, or if you find you are experiencing hunger, a second mid-morning detox shake can be added to your daily meal plan. Get started right away with one or more of these options that provide a healthy dose of protein during your detox:

Option #1

- 1 serving whey protein isolate, any flavor (or rice, hemp or vegan protein)
- 2 tablespoons ground flaxseed or chia seed or 1 serving of a fiber supplement (optional, but highly recommended)
- 1 tablespoon almond, hazelnut, cashew or pumpkin seed butter
- 1/4 teaspoon cinnamon
- 1/2–3/4 cup water or unsweetened almond milk
- 3–4 ice cubes (optional)
- Stevia (optional)

Place all ingredients in a blender and blend on high speed until smooth and creamy. Alternatively, you can toss all the ingredients, except the water, into a protein shaker cup. When you are ready for a snack, add the water, shake well and drink.

Option #2

- 1 serving whey protein isolate, any flavor (or rice, hemp or vegan protein)
- 1/2–3/4 cup water or unsweetened almond milk
- 1/2 cup blueberries
- 2 tablespoons ground flaxseed or chia seed or 1 serving of a fiber supplement (optional, but highly recommended)
- 3–4 ice cubes (optional)
- Stevia (optional)

Place all ingredients in a blender and blend on high speed until smooth and creamy.

Option #3

1   serving whey protein isolate, any flavor (or rice, hemp or vegan protein)
1   scoop Clear Recovery (Clear Medicine)
½–¾ cup water

Combine ingredients and drink. This is a great "on the go" option because it does not require a blender.

Option #4

½–¾ cup unsweetened almond milk
½   cup pitted fresh or frozen cherries
2   tablespoons ground flaxseed or chia seed or 1 serving of a fiber supplement (optional, but highly recommended)
3/4 cup Fage Total 0% plain Greek yogurt or goat milk yogurt

Place all ingredients in a blender and blend on high until smooth and creamy.

A note regarding nutritional information: The nutrition content per meal may vary depending on the brands of foods selected. You may also visit the Book Extras section for *The Supercharged Hormone Diet* on drnatashaturner.com for additional recipe options.

WEEK 1:
Detoxification
(Your Grain-free and Potato-free Week)

All foods that could trigger excess insulin release, spur inflammation or increase cravings are completely removed from your diet during this week.

Day 1

Breakfast (7 a.m. to 8 a.m.)
Easy Egg White and Goat Cheese Omelette (page 283)

Mid-morning Snack (10 a.m.) (optional)
Detox Shake (pages 231–32) mixed in water. Blending with ice is optional.

Lunch (12 p.m. to 1 p.m.)
Protein-topped Feta and Peach Salad (page 292)

Mid-afternoon Snack (3 p.m. to 4 p.m.)
Detox Shake (pages 231–32) mixed in water. Blending with ice is optional.

Dinner (6 p.m. to 8 p.m. at the latest)
Tomato Turkey Delight (page 303)

Bedtime (10 p.m. to 11 p.m. at the latest)

Day 2

Breakfast (7 a.m. to 8 a.m.)
Refreshing Berry-Peach Smoothie (page 281)

Mid-morning Snack (10 a.m.) (optional)
Detox Shake (pages 231–32) mixed in water. Blending with ice is optional.

Lunch (12 p.m. to 1 p.m.)
Goat Cheese, Pear and Pine Nut Spinach Salad (page 292)

Mid-afternoon Snack (3 p.m. to 4 p.m.)
Detox Shake (pages 231–32) mixed in water. Blending with ice is optional.

Dinner (6 p.m. to 8 p.m. at the latest)
Chicken Souvlaki (page 322) and salad

Bedtime (10 p.m. to 11 p.m. at the latest)

Day 3

Breakfast (7 a.m. to 8 a.m.)
Berry Quick Delight with goat yogurt (page 285)
(Substitute: 1 scoop of whey protein for ricotta)

Mid-morning Snack (10 a.m.) (optional)
Detox Shake (pages 231–32) mixed in water. Blending with ice is
optional.

Lunch (12 p.m. to 1 p.m.)
Roasted Beet, Orange, Walnut and Baby Arugula Salad (page 293)
(Substitute: raspberries for oranges)

Mid-afternoon Snack (3 p.m. to 4 p.m.)
Detox Shake (pages 231–32) mixed in water. Blending with ice is
optional.

Dinner (6 p.m. to 8 p.m. at the latest)
Tilapia with Fresh Tropical Salsa (page 305)

Bedtime (10 p.m. to 11 p.m. at the latest)

Day 4

Breakfast (7 a.m. to 8 a.m.)
Mediterranean Omelette (page 286)

Mid-morning Snack (10 a.m.)
Detox Shake (pages 231–32) mixed in water. Blending with ice is optional.

Lunch (12 p.m. to 1 p.m.)
Puréed Squash and Apple Soup (page 295)
(Substitute: 1 or 2 hard-boiled eggs for cottage cheese)

Mid-afternoon Snack (3 p.m. to 4 p.m.)
Detox Shake (pages 231–32) mixed in water. Blending with ice is optional.

Dinner (6 a.m. to 8 p.m. at the latest)
Roasted Chicken Breasts (page 313) with Cauliflower Mash (page 315).

Bedtime (10 p.m. to 11 p.m. at the latest)

Day 5

Breakfast (7 a.m. to 8 a.m.)
Power Protein Scramble (page 287)
(Substitute: goat cheese for cow's milk cheese)

Mid-morning Snack (10 a.m.)
Detox Shake (pages 231–32) mixed in water. Blending with ice is optional.

Lunch (12 p.m. to 1 p.m.)
Japanese Spinach Salad (page 296)

Mid-afternoon Snack (3 p.m. to 4 p.m.)
Detox Shake (pages 231–32) mixed in water. Blending with ice is optional.

Dinner (6 p.m. to 8 p.m. at the latest)
Pecan-crusted Chicken Breasts with Steamed Asparagus and Rapini (page 314)

Bedtime (10 p.m. to 11 p.m. at the latest)

Day 6

Breakfast (7 a.m. to 8 a.m.)
Easy Egg White and Goat Cheese Omelette (page 293)

Mid-morning Snack (10 a.m.)
Detox Shake (pages 231–32) mixed in water. Blending with ice is optional.

Lunch (12 p.m. to 1 p.m.)
Summer Raspberry Salad (page 296)

Mid-afternoon Snack (3 p.m. to 4 p.m.)
Detox Shake (pages 231–32) mixed in water. Blending with ice is optional.

Dinner (6 p.m. to 8 p.m. at the latest)
Perfect Pesto Chicken with Cauliflower Mash (page 315)

Bedtime (10 p.m. to 11 p.m. at the latest)

Day 7

Breakfast (7 a.m. to 8 a.m.)
Spanish Chicken Dish (page 291)

Mid-morning Snack (10 a.m.) (optional)
Detox Shake (pages 231–32) mixed in water. Blending with ice is optional.

Lunch (12 p.m. to 1 p.m.)
Roasted Vegetable Soup (page 298)
(Substitute: protein for goat milk yogurt or a hard-boiled egg)

Mid-afternoon Snack (3 p.m. to 4 p.m.)
Detox Shake (pages 231–32) mixed in water. Blending with ice is optional.

Dinner (6 p.m. to 8 p.m. at the latest)
Grilled Veggie and Sea Scallop Kebabs (page 317)

Bedtime (10 p.m. to 11 p.m. at the latest)

FOODS TO ENJOY

Grains and starchy vegetables: No foods in this category are allowed in week 1 of the detox

Unlimited vegetables: all vegetables except corn and potatoes

Fruits: all fruits except oranges, tangerines, grapefruit, dried fruits, raisins, dates, figs. Lemons and limes are permitted.

All beans (maximum 1 serving a day): lentils, black beans, kidney beans, mung beans, chickpeas

Two servings a day (2 tablespoons each) nuts and seeds: all nuts and seeds except peanuts and pistachios. Choices include cashews, walnuts, Brazil nuts, sesame seeds, pumpkin seeds, sunflower seeds, pecans, etc.

Fish and meat: all poultry (chicken, turkey, duck, etc.), fish and seafood

Two servings a day (1 tablespoon each) dairy: feta (made from sheep's or goat's milk), goat cheese, small amounts of butter; replace dairy milks with unsweetened almond, rice or soy milk

Soy products (1 serving a day): all soy products are fine unless you have experienced digestive upset (gas, bloating, indigestion or other symptoms) when you have eaten these products in the past. Choices include tofu, tempeh, soy nuts, soy milk and whole soybeans

Sweeteners: xylitol and stevia; maple syrup and honey should be used in your salad dressing only

Spices and condiments: all spices unless otherwise indicated; choices include cinnamon, cumin, dill, garlic, ginger, carob, oregano, parsley, rosemary, tarragon, thyme, turmeric, etc.

Oils and fats: canola oil, butter, flaxseed oil, hemp oil, coconut oil and extra-virgin olive oil are the only oils or added fats you should consume

Eggs: yolks and whites are fine

FOODS TO AVOID

All grains and potatoes: wheat, spelt, rye, kamut, barley. This means you will cut out bread, bagels, muffins, pastries, cakes, pasta, durum semolina, couscous, cookies, flour and cereals, millet, oats, rice and rice products, buckwheat, rice pasta, rice cakes, rice crackers, amaranth, slow-cooked oatmeal, sweet potato, white potato

Corn: popcorn, corn chips, fresh corn, canned corn

Citrus and processed fruits: oranges, grapefruit, tangerines, canned fruits, dried fruits including raisins, figs, dates, all other dried fruits

Beans: all beans are allowed, but if you want to be more conscious of your carbohydrate intake, reduce or avoid consumption of chickpeas and white beans

Nuts: peanuts, peanut butter, any products containing peanuts

Red meats: beef, pork, luncheon meats/cold cuts, sausage, bacon, lamb

Dairy: cow's milk cheeses, milk, yogurt, sour cream, soups and sauces containing dairy

Alcohol and caffeine: coffee, non-herbal tea, soft drinks, all alcoholic beverages

Sugar and artificial sweeteners: table sugar, any product with sugar added, rice syrup, high-fructose corn syrup, packaged foods, candies, soft drinks, juice and sweeteners like sucralose, aspartame and acesulfame-K.

Spices and condiments: chocolate, ketchup, mustard, relish, chutney, soy sauce, barbecue sauce, other store-bought condiments

Oils: hydrogenated oils, trans fatty acids, palm oil, soy oil, corn oil, cottonseed oil, vegetable oil, shortening, margarine; limit your intake of safflower and sunflower oils

WEEK 2:
Detoxification Continues
(1 daily serving of gluten-free grains
or potatoes is now permitted)

With week 1 of the *Supercharged* program under your belt, you have already begun to work wonders on your metabolism and hormonal health. For week 2 I include one grain or potato selection, but note that if you experience water retention, weight gain, cravings, increased hunger or fatigue after eating, it suggests that your body may not be ready to accept these types of carbohydrates yet. In this instance, there is no harm in repeating the week 1 plan, provided that you maintain your protein and healthy fat intake.

Although potatoes and gluten-free grains generally are hypoallergenic, they can cause these symptoms as a result of a sensitivity to the carbohydrates they contain. If you notice this reaction during this week, remove these sources of carbs again. You should also move on to my Carb Sensitivity Program after you have completed your 30-day *Supercharged* program help you to determine the best carbs for your metabolic and repair your ability to process carbs without weight gain.

Day 1

Breakfast (7 a.m. to 8 a.m.)
Mixed Berry and Pomegranate Smoothie (page 280)

Mid-morning Snack (10 a.m.) (optional)
Detox Shake (pages 231–32) mixed in water. Blending with ice is optional.

Lunch (12 p.m. to 1 p.m.)
Brie's Fresh and Easy Baby Spinach Salad (page 299)

Mid-afternoon Snack (3 p.m. to 4 p.m.)
Detox Shake (pages 231–32) mixed in water. Blending with ice is optional.

Dinner (6 p.m. to 8 p.m. at the latest)
Baked Halibut Topped with Broiled Tomato-Mango Salsa (page 318) (served with $1/2$ cup sweet potato or brown rice)

Bedtime (10 p.m. to 11 p.m. at the latest)

Day 2

Breakfast (7 a.m. to 8 a.m.)
Goat milk yogurt and Blueberry Smoothie (page 280)

Mid-morning Snack (10 a.m.)
Detox Shake (pages 231–32) mixed in water. Blending with ice is optional.

Lunch (12 p.m. to 1 p.m.)
Chicken Chili (page 319)

Mid-afternoon Snack (3 p.m. to 4 p.m.)
Detox Shake (pages 231–32) mixed in water. Blending with ice is optional.

Dinner (6 p.m. to 8 p.m. at the latest)
Chicken Cabbage Cashew Stir-fry (page 321)

Bedtime (10 p.m. to 11 p.m. at the latest)

Day 3

Breakfast (7 a.m. to 8 a.m.)
Scrambled Eggs with Dill and Feta Served on Sliced Tomatoes
(page 284)

Mid-morning Snack (10 a.m.)
Detox Shake (pages 231–32) mixed in water. Blending with ice is
optional.

Lunch (12 p.m. to 1 p.m.)
Summer Raspberry Salad (page 296)

Mid-afternoon Snack (3 p.m. to 4 p.m.)
Detox Shake (pages 231–32) mixed in water. Blending with ice is
optional.

Dinner (6 p.m. to 8 p.m. at the latest)
Halibut with Roasted Tomatoes (page 320) and $^1/_2$ cup rice.

Bedtime (10 p.m. to 11 p.m. at the latest)

Day 4

Breakfast (7 a.m. to 8 a.m.)
Heart's Delight Oatmeal and Banana Smoothie (page 281)

Mid-morning Snack (10 a.m.)
Detox Shake (pages 231–32) mixed in water. Blending with ice is optional.

Lunch (12 p.m. to 1 p.m.)
Japanese Spinach Salad (page 296)

Mid-afternoon Snack (3 p.m. to 4 p.m.)
Detox Shake (pages 231–32) mixed in water. Blending with ice is optional.

Dinner (6 p.m. to 8 p.m.at the latest)
Chicken Stir-fry with Peppers and Fresh Basil and basmati rice (page 307)

Bedtime (10 p.m. to 11 p.m. at the latest)

Day 5

Breakfast (7 a.m. to 8 a.m.)
Easy Egg White and Goat Cheese Omelette (page 283)

Mid-morning Snack (10 a.m.)
Detox Shake (pages 231–32) mixed in water. Blending with ice is optional.

Lunch (12 p.m. to 1 p.m.)
Puréed Squash and Apple Soup (page 295)
(Substitute: goat cheese for cottage cheese)

Mid-afternoon Snack (3 p.m. to 4 p.m.)
Detox Shake (pages 231–32) mixed in water. Blending with ice is optional.

Dinner (6 p.m. to 8 p.m. at the latest)
Chicken Souvlaki (page 322) with basmati rice

Bedtime (10 p.m. to 11 p.m. at the latest)

Day 6

Breakfast (7 a.m. to 8 a.m.)
Mediterranean Omelette (page 286)

Mid-morning Snack (10 a.m.)
Detox Shake (pages 231–32) mixed in water. Blending with ice is optional.

Lunch (12 p.m. to 1 p.m.)
Protein-topped Feta and Peach Salad (page 292)

Mid-afternoon Snack (3 p.m. to 4 p.m.)
Detox Shake (pages 231–32) mixed in water. Blending with ice is optional.

Dinner (6 p.m. to 8 p.m. at the latest)
Whole Roasted Chicken and Herb-baked Sweet Potato Fries (page 302)

Bedtime (10 p.m. to 11 p.m. at the latest)

Day 7

Breakfast (7 a.m. to 8 a.m.)
Dose of Dopamine Chocolate Yogurt (page 287)
(Substitute: goat yogurt for organic yogurt)

Mid-morning Snack (10 a.m.)
Detox Shake (pages 231–32) mixed in water. Blending with ice is optional.

Lunch (12 p.m. to 1 p.m.)
Brie's Fresh and Easy Baby Spinach Salad (use 1 tablespoon of feta instead of $^1/_2$ cup) (page 299)

Mid-afternoon Snack (3 p.m. to 4 p.m.)
Detox Shake (pages 231–32) mixed in water. Blending with ice is optional.

Dinner (6 p.m. to 8 p.m. at the latest)
Rice Pasta with Chicken, Goat Cheese and Roasted Asparagus (page 300)

Bedtime (10 p.m. to 11 p.m. at the latest)

Week 2: Summary of Your Foods to Enjoy and Avoid (1 serving of gluten-free grains or potatoes)

FOODS TO ENJOY

Gluten-free grains and potatoes: You may enjoy one ½-cup serving a day of gluten-free grains or potatoes, including millet, quinoa, buckwheat, rice and rice products, sweet potato, white potato. Remember to remove these foods if you experience weight gain, hunger or cravings.

Unlimited vegetables: all vegetables except for corn

Fruits: all fruits except for oranges, tangerines, grapefruit, dried fruits, raisins, dates, figs. Lemons and limes are permitted.

All beans (maximum 1 serving a day): lentils, black beans, kidney beans, mung beans, chickpeas

Two servings a day (2 tablespoons each) nuts and seeds: all nuts and seeds except peanuts. Choices include cashews, walnuts, Brazil nuts, sesame seeds, pumpkin seeds, sunflower seeds, pecans, etc.

Fish and meat: all poultry (chicken, turkey, duck, etc.), fish and seafood

Two servings a day (1 tablespoon each) dairy: feta (made from sheep's or goat's milk), goat cheese, small amounts of butter; replace dairy milks with unsweetened almond, rice or soy milk

Soy products (1 serving a day): all soy products are fine unless you have experienced digestive upset (gas, bloating, indigestion or other symptoms) when you have eaten these products in the past. Choices include tofu, tempeh, soy nuts, soy milk and whole soybeans

Sweeteners: xylitol and stevia; maple syrup and honey should be used in your salad dressing only

Spices and condiments: all spices unless otherwise indicated; choices include cinnamon, cumin, dill, garlic, ginger, carob, oregano, parsley, rosemary, tarragon, thyme, turmeric, etc.

Oils and fats: canola oil, butter, flaxseed oil, hemp oil, coconut oil and extra-virgin olive oil are the only oils or added fats you should consume

Eggs: yolks and whites are fine

FOODS TO AVOID

Grains containing gluten: wheat, spelt, rye, kamut, barley. This means you will cut out most breads, bagels, muffins, pastries, cakes, pastas, durum semolina, couscous, cookies, flours and cereals, oats, amaranth, slow-cooked oatmeal

Corn: popcorn, corn chips, fresh corn, canned corn

Citrus and processed fruits: oranges, grapefruit, tangerines, canned fruits, dried fruits including raisins, figs, dates, all other dried fruits

Beans: all beans are allowed, but if you want to be more conscious of your carbohydrate intake, reduce or avoid consumption of chickpeas and white beans

Nuts: peanuts, peanut butter, pistachios; any products containing peanuts or pistachios

Red meats: beef, pork, luncheon meats/cold cuts, sausage, bacon, lamb

Dairy: cow's milk cheeses, milk, yogurt, sour cream, soups and sauces containing dairy

Alcohol and caffeine: coffee, non-herbal tea, soft drinks, all alcoholic beverages

Sugar and artificial sweeteners: table sugar, any product with sugar added, rice syrup, high-fructose corn syrup, packaged foods, candies, soft drinks, juice and sweeteners like sucralose, Splenda, aspartame, etc.

Spices and condiments: chocolate, ketchup, mustard, relish, chutney, soy sauce, barbecue sauce, other store-bought condiments

Oils: hydrogenated oils, trans fatty acids, palm oil, soy oil, corn oil, cottonseed oil, vegetable oil, shortening, margarine; limit your intake of safflower and sunflower oils

WEEK 3:
The Transition from Step 1—Detox to Step 2—the Glyci-Med Nutrition Approach

Many of us with food sensitivities don't even realize how bad we feel until the problematic foods are removed from our diet. Then, suddenly, getting out of bed becomes easier; our energy, mood and concentration improve; and joint pain, headaches and sinus congestion disappear. During your anti-inflammatory detox, you will take these foods out of your diet for a specific period of time to give your body a break and a chance to calm down and detoxify.

Slowly reintroducing each food after a break can allow you to connect particular symptoms with your food choices. Once you have finished avoiding certain foods for the first 14 days of your detox, you will slowly reintroduce them. Often it's the end of a detox that's the most important part because it allows you to make the connection between certain foods and how they make you feel.

Reintroduce each food individually, one day at a time, as I have outlined in the meal plan starting on page 255. You will try the least allergenic foods first, followed by the foods with the greatest tendency to cause problems. Then you won't eat each test food again until you have introduced all the other foods. Because they are permitted in the next step of your diet, I recommend you test rye, kamut, cheese, yogurt and whole wheat, as long as your body likes them and remains symptom-free. When you reintroduce these foods, be on the lookout for symptoms that point to an allergy or intolerance. Check the chart on page 254 to see the most common reactions prompted by certain foods. I have also created a spot in your wellness tracker, in Part Three, for you to note any symptoms you may experience. It is certainly helpful to record how you feel on a daily basis.

General Guidelines for Your Food Reintroduction Process

1. You will reintroduce one new food each day and have the food one or two times on that day only. This means you will not try that food again until you have introduced all the other foods. Don't bother reintroducing foods you do not like. You will enter week 4 of the program sooner if you decide to skip one or more of the foods during the reintroduction process.

2. If you have a reaction to a food, it's up to you to decide if you would like to continue eating the food. Know that the reaction is the purpose of this process, and it will allow you to move forward to the Glyci-Med approach knowing which foods help you to look and feel your best.

3. Your shopping list for this process should include (simply leave out any item from this list you do not plan to test):

   - Grapefruit
   - Orange
   - Kamut—try kamut bread or kamut pasta (made by Sobaya)
   - Rye—100 percent rye bread, Wasa or Ryvita crispbread or Finn Crisp, Organic
   - Yogurt—plain organic yogurt and Greek yogurt
   - Cheese—reduced-fat Swiss, reduced-fat Jarlsberg, low-fat ricotta and/or pressed organic cottage cheese
   - Ezekiel products, such as Ezekiel bread from Food for Life, in the freezer or organic section

Keep in mind that the symptoms you should watch for are not only related to digestion. For example:

INTRODUCED FOOD	TYPICAL REACTIONS/SYMPTOMS
Wheat Whole-wheat pasta, bread, bagels, etc.	Gas, bloating, constipation, fatigue immediately after eating the food; fatigue on waking the next day or a gradual decline in energy noticed over the next week or so; irritability, anxiety, headaches, water retention (can't get your rings off, puffiness under the eyes the next day); dark circles under the eyes on waking the next day
Citrus Oranges, grapefruit, etc.	Excess mucus, stomach upset, headaches or migraines
Kamut Kamut bread or pasta	Similar to wheat
Rye Rye bread, Wasa or Ryvita crispbreads	Similar to wheat
Corn Corn kernels, organic popcorn, organic blue corn chips	Gas, bloating, headaches, constipation
Dairy Plain organic yogurt first Next introduce low-fat cheese or plain organic cottage cheese	Gas, bloating, constipation, diarrhea, sinus congestion, post-nasal drip, constant need to clear your throat, allergies (environmental) may worsen
Red meat Introduce beef, lamb and pork separately if you wish	Joint pain, constipation, indigestion
Sugar, alcohol and caffeine (coffee, regular tea); try these only after you have introduced all the other foods	Headaches, fatigue, water retention, increased hunger or cravings

Day 1—Citrus

Breakfast (7 a.m. to 8 a.m.)
Grapefruit with 1 serving goat milk yogurt

Mid-morning Snack (10 a.m.)
Detox Shake (pages 231–32) mixed in water. Blending with ice is optional.

Lunch (12 p.m. to 1 p.m.)
Roasted Beet, Orange, Walnut and Baby Arugula Salad (page 293)

Mid-afternoon Snack (3 p.m. to 4 p.m.)
Detox Shake (pages 231–32) mixed in water. Blending with ice is optional.

Dinner (6 p.m. to 8 p.m. at the latest)
Rice Pasta with Chicken, Goat Cheese and Roasted Asparagus (page 300)

Bedtime (10 p.m. to 11 p.m. at the latest)

Day 2—Yogurt

Breakfast (7 a.m. to 8 a.m.)
Dose of Dopamine Chocolate Yogurt (page 287)

Mid-morning Snack (10 a.m.)
Detox Shake (pages 231–32) mixed in water. Blending with ice is optional.

Lunch (12 p.m. to 1 p.m.)
Puréed Squash and Apple Soup (page 295)
(Substitute: 2 tablespoons of organic yogurt for cottage cheese)

Mid-afternoon Snack (3 p.m. to 4 p.m.)
Detox Shake (pages 231–32) mixed in water. Blending with ice is optional.

Dinner (6 p.m. to 8 p.m. at the latest)
Whole Roasted Chicken and Herb-baked Sweet Potato Fries (page 302)

Bedtime (10 p.m. to 11 p.m. at the latest)

Day 3—Cheese

Breakfast (7 a.m. to 8 a.m.)
Berry Flax Cottage Cheese (page 288)

Mid-morning Snack (10 a.m.)
Detox Shake (pages 231–32) mixed in water. Blending with ice is
optional.

Lunch (12 p.m. to 1 p.m.)
Low-fat Caesar Salad with Grilled Chicken or Shrimp (page 297)
(substitute: no-fat yogurt for goat milk yogurt)

Mid-afternoon Snack (3 p.m. to 4 p.m.)
Detox Shake (pages 231–32) mixed in water. Blending with ice is
optional.

Dinner (6 p.m. to 8 p.m. at the latest)
Carb-conscious Lasagna (page 304)

Bedtime (10 p.m. to 11 p.m. at the latest)

Day 4—Rye

Breakfast (7 a.m. to 8 a.m.)
One hard-boiled egg and one slice of 100% rye bread (must not contain wheat flour) topped with almond butter

Mid-morning Snack (10 a.m.)
Detox Shake (pages 231–32) mixed in water. Blending with ice is optional.

Lunch (12 p.m. to 1 p.m.)
Wasa crisps topped with goat cheese; sliced tomatoes and Roasted Vegetable Soup (page 298)

Mid-afternoon Snack (3 p.m. to 4 p.m.)
Detox Shake (pages 231–32) mixed in water. Blending with ice is optional.

Dinner (6 p.m. to 8 p.m. at the latest)
Tomato Turkey Delight (page 303)

Bedtime (10 p.m. to 11 p.m. at the latest)

Day 5—Kamut

Breakfast (7 a.m. to 8 a.m.)
Scrambled Eggs with Dill and Feta Served on Sliced Tomatoes (page 284)

Mid-morning Snack (10 a.m.)
Detox Shake (pages 231–32) mixed in water. Blending with ice is optional.

Lunch (12 p.m. to 1 p.m.)
Kamut bread toasted with nitrate-free sliced turkey, mayo and tomatoes

Mid-afternoon Snack (3 p.m. to 4 p.m.)
Detox Shake (pages 231–32) mixed in water. Blending with ice is optional.

Dinner (6 p.m. to 8 p.m. at the latest)
Kamut Pasta with Peas and Ricotta (page 301)
(Substitute: goat cheese for ricotta cheese)

Bedtime (10 p.m. to 11 p.m. at the latest)

Day 6—Ezekiel Products

Breakfast (7 a.m. to 8 a.m.)
Sunday French Toast (page 288)

Mid-morning Snack (10 a.m.)
Detox Shake (pages 231–32) mixed in water. Blending with ice is optional.

Lunch (12 p.m. to 1 p.m.)
Tasty Toasted Tuna Salad (page 299)
(substitute: $1/2$ can of tuna for the cottage cheese)

Mid-afternoon Snack (3 p.m. to 4 p.m.)
Detox Shake (pages 231–32) mixed in water. Blending with ice is optional.

Dinner (6 p.m. to 8 p.m. at the latest)
Chicken Stir-fry with Peppers and Fresh Basil (page 307)

Bedtime (10 p.m. to 11 p.m. at the latest)

Day 7—Whole Wheat

Breakfast (7 a.m. to 8 a.m.)
Refreshing Berry-Peach Smoothie (page 281)

Mid-morning Snack (10 a.m.)
Detox Shake (pages 231–32) mixed in water. Blending with ice is optional.

Lunch (12 p.m. to 1 p.m.)
Tasty Egg and Cheese Sandwich (using goat cheese) (page 286) and mixed greens
(substitute: wheat bread for the rye bread)

Mid-afternoon Snack (3 p.m. to 4 p.m.)
Detox Shake (pages 231–32) mixed in water. Blending with ice is optional.

Dinner (6 p.m. to 8 p.m. at the latest)
Rice Pasta with Chicken, Goat Cheese and Roasted Asparagus (page 300) (Substitute: whole-wheat pasta for rice pasta)

Bedtime (10 p.m. to 11 p.m. at the latest)

WEEK 4:
The Glyci-Med Approach

You are now ready to transition from a diet that focused on detoxification and the identification of food allergies to one that centers on eating for glycemic (and hormonal) balance. By now you will likely have lost all of your cravings and anywhere from 3 to 12 pounds! You might also notice improved digestion, more restful sleep, increased energy, better focus and glowing skin.

The detox is an essential step to restore your wellness and to create the foundation of a diet to help you look and feel your best every day. Most importantly, eating for blood sugar and insulin balance will keep you strong, lean and operating like a finely tuned machine. This philosophy of eating will also work to keep your cholesterol low, blood pressure controlled and reduce your risk of heart disease, diabetes, Alzheimer's disease and certain types of cancer.

The delicious and satisfying meals laid out here contain all of the needed elements to power up your fat-burning hormones. You will continue to have three meals and two snacks a day. At the end of week 4, your detox shake will be finished. You are free to replace it with any of the snack options I have listed for you in Chapter 10.

In the summary of your foods to enjoy and avoid for this week, presented at the end of the meal plan, you will notice some of the foods you were allowed during week 1 are no longer recommended. This is recommended because some foods that are hypoallergenic and anti-inflammatory are not necessarily low glycemic. Only those options that are low glycemic are recommended from this stage onward. For instance, rice pasta was allowed during the second week of your detox diet because it is hypoallergenic and gluten-free. Since rice pasta is, however, high glycemic, it is now no longer listed as a food to enjoy. If you plan to continue eating gluten-free, opt for grain selections and starchy carb products that are higher in fiber, such as sweet potatoes, millet or buckwheat.

At this point you should continue to lose 1 to 3 pounds per week and remain craving-free. If you find this not to be your case, I normally suggest many on to my Carb Sensitivity Program.

Also note that I have identified your best low-fat protein selections with a (**P**), your best low-GI carb selections with a (**C**) and your healthy fat selections with an (**F**). Remember, you have to select **one** from each category at every meal and snack, just as I have done for you in all the meal plans. The Carb Sensitivity Program will help you to determine if all of the starchy carb options permitted in the phase are actually suitable to your metabolism for ongoing weight loss. My philosophy is don't think no–carb but rather think about consuming the right carb for you! Not all "good" carbs are "good" for everyone. Our ability to metabolize candy is just as unique as our food sensitivities.

Day 1

Breakfast (7 a.m. to 8 a.m.)
Scrambled Eggs with Dill and Feta Served on Sliced Tomatoes (page 284)

Mid-morning Snack (10 a.m.)
Detox Shake (pages 231–32) mixed in water. Blending with ice is optional.

Lunch (12 p.m. to 1 p.m.)
Satisfying Serotonin Delight (page 290)

Mid-afternoon Snack (3 p.m. to 4 p.m.)
Detox Shake (pages 231–32) mixed in water. Blending with ice is optional.

Dinner (6 p.m. to 8 p.m. at the latest)
Curried Ginger Chicken Breast with Quinoa (page 306)

Bedtime (10 p.m. to 11 p.m. at the latest)

Day 2

Breakfast (7 a.m. to 8 a.m.)
Cottage or Ricotta Cheese Oatmeal Pancakes (page 282)

Mid-morning Snack (10 a.m.)
Detox Shake (pages 231–32) mixed in water. Blending with ice is optional.

Lunch (12 p.m. to 1 p.m.)
Spanish Chicken Dish (page 291)

Mid-afternoon Snack (3 p.m. to 4 p.m.)
Detox Shake (pages 231–32) mixed in water. Blending with ice is optional.

Dinner (6 p.m. to 8 p.m. at the latest)
Chicken Stir-fry with Peppers and Fresh Basil (page 307)

Bedtime (10 p.m. to 11 p.m. at the latest)

Day 3

Breakfast (7 a.m. to 8 a.m.)
Easy Egg White and Goat Cheese Omelette (page 283)
(Substitute: any low-fat cheese)

Mid-morning Snack (10 a.m.)
Detox Shake (pages 231–32) mixed in water. Blending with ice is
optional.

Lunch (12 p.m. to 1 p.m.)
Protein-topped Feta and Peach Salad (page 292)

Mid-afternoon Snack (3 p.m. to 4 p.m.)
Detox Shake (pages 231–32) mixed in water. Blending with ice is
optional.

Dinner (6 p.m. to 8 p.m. at the latest)
Mediterranean Chicken Kebabs with Greek Dipping Sauce (page 308)

Bedtime (10 p.m. to 11 p.m. at the latest)

Day 4

Breakfast (7 a.m. to 8 a.m.)
Berry Flax Cottage Cheese (page 288)

Mid-morning Snack (10 a.m.)
Detox Shake (pages 231–32) mixed in water. Blending with ice is optional.

Lunch (12 p.m. to 1 p.m.)
Easy Egg White and Goat Cheese Omelette (page 283)

Mid-afternoon Snack (3 p.m. to 4 p.m.)
Detox Shake (pages 231–32) mixed in water. Blending with ice is optional.

Dinner (6 p.m. to 8 p.m. at the latest)
Almond-crusted Chicken Breasts with Herbed New Potatoes and Baby Arugula Salad (page 309)

Bedtime (10 p.m. to 11 p.m. at the latest)

Day 5

Breakfast (7 a.m. to 8 a.m.)
Berry Quick Delight (page 285)

Mid-morning Snack (10 a.m.)
Detox Shake (pages 231–32) mixed in water. Blending with ice is optional.

Lunch (12 p.m. to 1 p.m.)
Low-fat Caesar Salad with Grilled Chicken or Shrimp (page 297)

Mid-afternoon Snack (3 p.m. to 4 p.m.)
Detox Shake (pages 231–32) mixed in water. Blending with ice is optional.

Dinner (6 p.m. to 8 p.m. at the latest)
Coconut Chicken Curry with Rice (page 310)

Bedtime (10 p.m. to 11 p.m. at the latest)

Day 6

Breakfast (7 a.m. to 8 a.m.)
Frozen Blueberry Yogurt (page 285)

Mid-morning Snack (10 a.m.)
Detox Shake (pages 231–32) mixed in water. Blending with ice is optional.

Lunch (12 p.m. to 1 p.m.)
Roasted Vegetable Soup (page 298)

Mid-afternoon Snack (3 p.m. to 4 p.m.)
Detox Shake (pages 231–32) mixed in water. Blending with ice is optional.

Dinner (6 p.m. to 8 p.m. at the latest)
Curried Shrimp (page 311)

Bedtime (10 p.m. to 11 p.m. at the latest)

Day 7

Breakfast (7 a.m. to 8 a.m.)
Power Protein Scramble (page 287)

Mid-morning Snack (10 a.m.)
Detox Shake (pages 231–32) mixed in water. Blending with ice is optional.

Lunch (12 p.m. to 1 p.m.)
Brie's Fresh and Easy Baby Spinach Salad (page 299)

Mid-afternoon Snack (3 p.m. to 4 p.m.)
Detox Shake (pages 231–32) mixed in water. Blending with ice is optional.

Dinner (6 p.m. to 8 p.m. at the latest)
Tilapia (page 305) served with Sweet Potato Pancakes (page 312)

Bedtime (10 p.m. to 11 p.m. at the latest)

WEEK 4: SUMMARY OF YOUR FOODS TO ENJOY AND AVOID

FOODS TO ENJOY AND SUGGESTED SERVING SIZES

C: Grains, starchy veggies and selected beans—1 serving per day:

Carrots, cooked	$^1/_2$ cup
Soybeans/edamame, shelled	$^1/_2$ cup
Summer squash	1 cup
Baby carrots, raw	$^1/_2$ cup
Beets, sliced	$^1/_2$ cup
Celery root (celeriac)	1 cup
Spaghetti squash	1 cup
Peas	$^1/_2$ cup
Ezekiel Sprouted Grain cereal	$^1/_3$ cup
Fiber One cereal	$^1/_2$ cup
All-Bran Bran Buds cereal	$^1/_3$ cup
Ezekiel bread	1 slice
Ezekiel wrap	1 wrap
Ezekiel English muffin	1 muffin
Kavli Crispy Thin Crispbread	3 pieces
Finn Crisp crispbread	1 slice
Ryvita Crispbread (Sunflower Seeds and Oats; Multigrain; Sesame; Dark Rye; Original)	4 crackers
Bulgur	$^1/_2$ cup
Buckwheat groats/kasha	$^1/_2$ cup
Rye bread	1 slice
Quinoa	$^1/_2$ cup
Winter squashes (acorn and butternut)	1 cup
Lima beans	$^1/_2$ cup

FOODS TO AVOID

C: Grains and starchy veggies—except for your cheat meal once a week:

White bread

White pasta

White rice

Bagels

Muffins

Pastries and pies

Cookies

Anything labeled as an "energy" bar

Spelt products (they tend to be lower in fiber than kamut)

Crackers

Granola bars

Sesame snacks

C: Grains, starchy veggies and selected beans—1 serving per day (continued from page 271):

Chickpeas (garbanzo beans)	$^1/_2$ cup
White beans	$^1/_2$ cup
Oat bran	$^1/_2$ cup
Adzuki beans	$^1/_2$ cup
Pinto beans	$^1/_2$ cup
Potatoes, boiled, or new potatoes	1 medium
Oatmeal, measured dry	$^1/_3$ cup
Steel-cut oats	$^1/_4$ cup
Kamut pasta	$^1/_2$ cup
Sweet potato, without skin	$^1/_2$ cup
Brown rice	$^1/_2$ cup
Basmati rice	$^1/_4$ cup
Whole-wheat pasta	$^1/_2$ cup
Pearl barley	$^1/_2$ cup

P/C/F: Nuts: (1 to 2 servings a day):

Walnuts	8
Cashews	6
Almonds	12
Seeds	2–3 tablespoons
Pistachios	20
Nut butter, preferably almond butter or organic peanut butter	1 tablespoon

C: Vegetables (unlimited):

All green vegetables, peppers, tomatoes, eggplant, zucchini, cauliflower, onions, leeks, artichokes, etc.

P/C/F: Nuts (except for your cheat meal once a week):

Peanuts

C: Vegetables (except for your cheat meal once a week):

Corn, parsnips

FOODS TO ENJOY AND SUGGESTED SERVINGS

C/P: Beans (1 serving per day—optional):

Calico beans	¹/₂ cup
Broad beans (fava beans)	¹/₂ cup
Cannellini beans	¹/₂ cup
Lentils	¹/₂ cup
Split peas	¹/₂ cup
Great Northern beans	¹/₂ cup
Mung beans	¹/₂ cup
Black beans	¹/₂ cup
Butter beans	¹/₂ cup
Kidney beans	¹/₂ cup
Navy beans	¹/₂ cup

C: Fruits (2 to 3 servings per day)

Cherries	15
Apricots	3
Prunes	3
Berries	1 cup
Peaches	1 small
Pears	1 small
Apples	1 small
Plums	1 small
Oranges	1 small
Kiwi	1 small
Grapefruit	1 whole
Watermelon	1 cup
Banana	¹/₂, in protein shakes only

FOODS TO AVOID

C: Fruits (except for your cheat meal once a week and in one smoothie a day):

Melons (cantaloupe, honeydew, etc.)
Dates
Raisins
Pineapple
Papaya
Mango
Grapes

FOODS TO ENJOY AND SUGGESTED SERVINGS

P: Proteins—3 to 4 servings, the size and width of your palm (3 to 4 oz for women/ 5–6 oz for men or the suggested size listed here):

Chicken, turkey	
Shellfish, fish	
Egg whites	$^2/_3$ cup (or 4 to 5 egg whites)
Eggs	2 whole, or 3 egg whites and 1 whole egg
Tofu or tempeh	8 oz
Cottage cheese or ricotta	$^1/_2$ cup for a snack, $^3/_4$ cup for a meal
Organic pressed cottage cheese	$^1/_2$ cup for a meal
Cabot 75% less fat (Cheddar)	2 servings = 18 g of protein
Fage Total 0% Greek yogurt, plain	6 oz = 18 g o f protein
Fage Total classic Greek yogurt, plain	7 oz = 18 g of protein
Lean red meat (preferably organic/grass fed)	1 serving
F/C/P: Dairy and substitutes (1 serving per day):	
Plain soy milk (unsweetened)	$^1/_2$ cup
Almond milk (unsweetened)	$^3/_4$ cup
Goat milk feta, goat cheese, sheep's-milk cheese	2 tablespoons
Goat milk yogurt	$^1/_2$ cup

FOODS TO AVOID

P: Proteins:

Luncheon meats or cold cuts

Sausage

Bacon

Marbled meats

Deep-fried foods

F/C/P: Dairy and substitutes (except for your cheat meal once a week):

Full-fat dairy products

Sour cream, ice cream

Rice milk

FOODS TO ENJOY AND SUGGESTED SERVINGS

F: Oils—3 to 4 servings per day:

Extra-virgin olive oil; must have **daily**	1 tablespoon
Avocado	$1/8$ to $1/4$ of a medium-size fruit
Mayonnaise, canola- or olive oil–based	1 teaspoon
Olives	5–6
Butter	1 teaspoon
Flaxseed, ground	1–3 tablespoons
Omega-3 egg yolks	1 for women; 2 for men
Organic coconut butter/oil	1 tablespoon

Spices and Condiments:

All spices are allowed unless otherwise indicated. For example, cinnamon, cumin, dill, garlic, ginger, carob, oregano, parsley, rosemary, tarragon, thyme, turmeric, etc.

Mustards and hot sauce, without sugar added

Drinks:

Sodium-free soda water

All herbal teas

Reverse-osmosis water is preferred.

Pure fruit juices should be limited to smoothies or mixed $1/4$ cup juice to $3/4$ cup water or sparkling water.

Organic coffee—maximum 1 cup per day, before noon and preferably before your workout, without sugar or sweeteners

FOODS TO AVOID
F: Oils:
Hydrogenated oils and trans fatty acids
Palm oil
Flaxseed oil
Soy oil
Corn oil
Cottonseed oil
Vegetable oil, shortening and all margarines
Limit your intake of safflower and sunflower oils.
Spices and Condiments (except for your cheat meal once a week):
Ketchup
Relish
Pickles with sugar added
Honey, maple syrup
Chutney
Soy sauce
Jams, jellies
Barbecue sauce or any other condiments containing sugar
Foods or drinks containing these products:
Avoid anything containing sugar, except for your one cheat meal a week
Alcohol—maximum 4 drinks a week
Diet soft drinks and juices containing artificial sweeteners

RECIPES

Breakfast Recipes

Mixed Berry and Pomegranate Smoothie (Serves 2)

- 2 servings whey protein isolate
- 1 cup frozen mixed berries
- $^1/_4$ cup unsweetened pomegranate juice (preferably POM)
- 2 tablespoons almond butter
- $^1/_4$ cup water
- $^1/_4$ cup ice cubes

Combine all the ingredients in a blender and purée on high speed until smooth.

Calories 252 | Protein 28 g | Fat 10 g | Carbohydrates 16 g | Fiber 4 g

Goat Milk Yogurt and Blueberry Smoothie (Serves 1)

- 1 serving whey protein isolate
- $^1/_2$ cup plain goat milk yogurt
- $^1/_2$ frozen banana
- $^1/_2$ cup frozen blueberries
- 1 tablespoon chia seeds
- $^1/_2$ cup water

Combine all the ingredients in a blender and purée on high speed until smooth.

Calories 326 | Protein 32 g | Fat 8 g | Carbohydrates 25 g | Fiber 7 g

Refreshing Berry-Peach Smoothie (Serves 1)

- 1 serving whey protein isolate
- 1 whole ripe peach, peeled, pitted and sliced (or approximately $^3/_4$ to 1 cup frozen peach slices)
- $^1/_2$ cup frozen strawberries
- $^3/_4$ cup unsweetened almond milk (preferably Almond Breeze) or soy milk (preferably Eden Foods Edensoy)
- 1 tablespoon chia seeds
- $^1/_2$ cup ice cubes

Combine all the ingredients in a blender and purée on high speed until smooth.

Calories 276 | Protein 29 g | Fat 8 g | Carbohydrates 33 g | Fiber 10 g

Heart's Delight Oatmeal and Banana Smoothie (Serves 1)

- $^1/_4$ cup old-fashioned, slow-cooked oats (preferably McCann's Steel Cut Oats)
- $^1/_4$ teaspoon cinnamon
- $^1/_4$ cup plain goat milk yogurt
- $^1/_2$ banana, sliced
- $^1/_2$ cup unsweetened almond milk (preferably Almond Breeze) or soy milk (preferably Eden Foods Edensoy)
- $^1/_2$ serving whey protein isolate

Combine all the ingredients in a blender and purée on high speed until smooth.

Calories 296 | Protein 21 g | Fat 6 g | Carbohydrates 29 g | Fiber 3 g

Cottage or Ricotta Cheese Oatmeal Pancakes (Serves 2)

- 1 cup old-fashioned, slow-cooked oats (preferably McCann's Steel Cut Oats)
- 1 tablespoon ground flaxseed or ground chia seed
- $^1/_4$ cup fresh blueberries
- $^1/_2$ cup low-fat cottage cheese or ricotta cheese
- 6 egg whites or $^3/_4$ cup egg whites
- $^1/_2$ teaspoon pure vanilla extract
- 2 teaspoons coconut oil

Combine the cooked oats and ground seeds in a large bowl. Stir in the blueberries, cheese, egg whites and vanilla extract.

Heat 1 teaspoon of the oil in a large skillet over medium heat. Pour $^1/_4$ cup of the pancake mixture into two areas on the pan. Cook until bubbles appear on the top of the batter and the edges appear set. Flip the pancakes and cook until set in the center. Repeat using the other teaspoon of oil.

If desired, top with 2 teaspoons of Eden Organic Apple Butter or $^1/_4$ cup fresh berries.

Calories 318 | Protein 24 g | Fat 10 g | Carbohydrates 34 g | Fiber 7 g

Easy Egg White and Goat Cheese Omelette (Serves 2)

- 10   egg whites or 1 1/4 cups egg whites
- 2   egg yolks (omega-3 eggs) or 1/4 avocado, sliced
  Salt and pepper to taste
- 2   teaspoons extra-virgin olive oil
- 2   heaping tablespoons goat cheese
- 4–6   tablespoons sugar-free prepared salsa
- 1   cup apple, chopped

Whisk the egg whites (and yolks, if included in the recipe) and season with salt and pepper. In a small skillet, heat 1 teaspoon of the oil and pour in half the egg mixture. Cook while pulling the egg mixture to the side of the pan, allowing the runny part to flow underneath until set (about 2 to 3 minutes). Top with half of the cheese and salsa (and sliced avocado, if using). Gently slide the omelette onto a plate, tipping the pan to fold the omelette. Repeat using the other teaspoon of oil. Enjoy with the chopped apple on the side.

(Note that this meal can be enjoyed with cow's milk cheese instead of goat cheese *after* the first 2 weeks of your detox. In this case, you can add 2 slices of low-fat Swiss or Jarlsberg cheese.)

Calories 250 | Protein 27 g | Fat 11 g | Carbohydrates 11 g | Fiber 2 g

Scrambled Eggs with Dill and Feta Served on Sliced Tomatoes (Serves 1)

- 4 egg whites and 1 whole egg (skip the whole egg if you double the feta)
- 1 ounce goat feta cheese (use 2 ounces if you skip the additional egg)
- 1 small tomato, sliced
- 1 tablespoon chopped fresh dill for garnish
  Salt and pepper to taste

Whisk the egg whites (and whole egg if included) in a bowl and add pepper. Stir the cheese into the egg mixture.

Heat the oil in a small skillet. Add the eggs and mix them in the pan with a wooden spatula until set.

Place 2 to 3 large tomato slices on a plate, pile the eggs on top of the tomatoes, sprinkle with the dill and enjoy. Can add a mixed green salad for a tasty low-calorie, low-carb meal.

Calories 221 | Protein 25 g | Fat 11 g | Carbohydrates 6 g | Fiber 1 g

Delicious Apple Dish (Serves 1)

- $^1/_3$ cup old-fashioned, slow-cooking oats (preferably McCann's Steel Cut Oats)
- $^1/_2$ cup milk (almond, soy, hemp or low-fat 1% cow's milk)
- $^1/_2$ Granny Smith apple, chopped
- 1 serving whey protein isolate (vanilla)
  Cinnamon or maple extract to taste
- 1 tablespoon slivered almonds

On the stove top, boil $^3/_4$ cup of water and cook the oatmeal. Add the milk. Mix in the apple, protein powder, cinnamon or maple extract and almonds. Enjoy!

Calories 330 | Protein 33 g | Fat 10 g | Carbohydrates 28 g | Fiber 5 g

Berry Quick Delight (Serves 1)

- $1/2$ cup blueberries, raspberries, blackberries or a berry mixture
- $1/2$ cup plain Fage total classic Greek yogurt or goat milk yogurt
- $1/2$ cup low-fat ricotta cheese
  Lemon or vanilla extract to taste
- 1 packet stevia (optional)
- 1 tablespoon sliced almonds

Blend together the berries, yogurt, ricotta cheese, flavoring and stevia. Sprinkle with the almonds.

Calories 267 | Protein 28 g | Fat 9 g | Carbohydrates 22 g | Fiber 4 g

Frozen Blueberry Yogurt (Serves 1)

- $1/2$ cup Fage total classic Greek yogurt, plain
- $3/4$ cup frozen blueberries, strawberries, raspberries or blackberries
- $1/2$ cup low-fat cottage cheese or ricotta cheese
- 1 tablespoon almond butter
- 1 packet stevia (optional)

Combine all the ingredients in a blender or food processor and blend until smooth.

Calories 318 | Protein 30 g | Fat 10 g | Carbohydrates 28 g | Fiber 5 g

Mediterranean Omelette (Serves 1)

4   egg whites or $1/2$ cup liquid egg whites
4   sliced black or green olives
2   slices nitrate-, and sulfite-free deli-style turkey slices, chopped
     (if you prefer to omit the turkey, increase to 6 egg whites)
1   ounce low-fat Swiss or Jarlsberg cheese or goat cheese
$1/2$ cup mixed berries

In a non-stick pan, cook the egg whites until slightly set. Add the olives, turkey and your choice of cheese. Once set, fold over and heat until cooked. Enjoy with $1/2$ cup of berries on the side.

Calories 204 | Protein 22 g | Fat 8 g | Carbohydrates 12 g | Fiber 2 g

Tasty Egg and Cheese Sandwich (Serves 1)

1   tomato, sliced
3   egg whites plus 1 egg, scrambled
1   slice reduced-fat Swiss or Jarlsberg or Cabot 75% less fat
     Cheddar or 1 tablespoon low-fat goat cheese
2   slices 100% rye bread, toasted, or organic Finn Crisp
     Fresh dill, chopped

Pile the tomato slices, eggs, and cheese on the slices of toast or crisp. Sprinkle with the dill and enjoy.

Calories 289 | Protein 26 g | Fat 9 g | Carbohydrates 28 g | Fiber 6 g

Power Protein Scramble (Serves 1)

- 2 teaspoons extra-virgin olive oil
- $1/4$ cup chopped red onion
- $1/2$ cup chopped red pepper
  - Garlic salt and pepper to taste
- 4 egg whites or $1/2$ cup liquid egg whites
- 1 ounce Cabot 75% less fat Cheddar

Place a skillet over medium heat and heat the olive oil. Sauté the onion and pepper until just tender, about 3 to 5 minutes. Add the garlic salt and pepper.

In a bowl, whisk the egg whites and pour into the pan over the veggie mixture. Cook, stirring, until the eggs are scrambled and set. Place the mixture on a plate and top with the cheese.

Calories 255 | Protein 25 g | Fat 12 g | Carbohydrates 12 g | Fiber 3 g

Dose of Dopamine Chocolate Yogurt (Serves 1)

- 1 tablespoon organic unsweetened cocoa powder (preferably Green & Black's)
- 1 cup Fage total classic Greek yogurt, plain
- $3/4$ serving whey protein isolate (vanilla or chocolate)
- 1 tablespoon chopped nuts (preferably walnuts, pecans or almonds)

Stir all the ingredients together and enjoy.

Calories 241 | Protein 25 g | Fat 9 g | Carbohydrates 22 g | Fiber 3 g

Sunday French Toast (Serves 1)

2 egg whites

$^1/_2$ serving whey protein isolate

1 teaspoon coconut oil

1 $^1/_2$ slices Cinnamon Raisin Ezekiel Bread

Cinnamon to taste

Mix the egg and whey protein isolate in a bowl. Heat the coconut oil in a skillet. Dip the bread in the egg mixture and fry. You may top this with cinnamon and 1 tablespoon of plain nonfat yogurt or low-fat cottage cheese.

Calories 246 | Protein 25 g | Fat 7 g | Carbohydrates 24 g | Fiber 4 g

Berry Flax Cottage Cheese (Serves 1)

$^3/_4$ cup low-fat ricotta or cottage cheese

$^1/_2$ cup strawberries

$^1/_2$ cup blueberries

1 tablespoon ground flaxseed or chia seeds

1 tablespoon chopped almonds

Mix the cheese, strawberries and blueberries in a bowl. Sprinkle the ground flaxseed or chia seeds and almonds over top.

Calories 307 | Protein 27 g | Fat 11 g | Carbohydrates 26 g | Fiber 6 g

High-Protein Breakfast Muffin (Serves 1)

- 1 teaspoon extra-virgin olive oil
- 2 egg whites
  Salt and pepper to taste
- $^1/_2$ Ezekiel English muffin
- 2 ounces Cabot 75% less fat Cheddar or reduced fat Swiss or Jarlsberg

Heat the oil in a skillet and cook the egg whites. Add the salt and pepper to taste. Meanwhile, toast the English muffin and top with the cheese. Place the cooked egg mixture on the toasted muffin. Enjoy with berries or apple on the side.

Calories 302 | Protein 33 g | Fat 8 g | Carbohydrates 24 g | Fiber 4 g

High-Protein Breakfast Muffin

Savory Sprouted Grain Breakfast (Serves 1)

- $^1/_4$ cup Ezekiel Sprouted Grain cereal
- 1 cup unsweetened almond milk
- 1 tablespoon hemp hearts
- $^3/_4$ serving whey protein isolate (vanilla)
- 1 tablespoon Fage total 0% Greek yogurt, plain

Combine the cereal, milk, hemp hearts and whey protein isolate in a bowl or blend well in a blender. Top with the yogurt and enjoy.

Calories 292 | Protein 27 g | Fat 11 g | Carbohydrates 27 g | Fiber 5 g

Savory Sprouted Grain Breakfast

Satisfying Serotonin Delight (Serves 1)

- 1 cup 100% pure pumpkin (canned), no salt or sugar added
- 1 serving whey protein isolate (vanilla)
- 1/2 teaspoon cinnamon
- 1 tablespoon chopped pecans

Stir all the ingredients together and enjoy.

Calories 298 | Protein 28 g | Fat 13 g | Carbohydrates 24 g | Fiber 8 g

Strawberry Shortcake Pancakes (Serves 1)

- 4 egg whites (or 1/2 cup of liquid egg whites)
- 1/3 cup dry oatmeal
- 1 teaspoon slivered or chopped almonds
- 1/2 serving whey protein isolate (vanilla or strawberry)
- 1 teaspoon olive or coconut oil
- 4–6 fresh strawberries, sliced
  Dash of cinnamon

Combine the egg whites, oatmeal, almonds and whey protein isolate in a bowl. Heat the oil in a skillet, and cook the egg mixture until you see bubbles on the top of the pancake. Flip and cook until set. Remove from the pan, top with the berries and cinnamon. If desired, add a few tablespoons of plain organic yogurt to the berries and sweeten with stevia.

Calories 301 | Protein 31 g | Fat 8 g | Carbohydrates 27 g | Fiber 5 g

Lunch Recipes
Spanish Chicken Dish (Serves 2)

1 1/2 tablespoons extra-virgin olive oil or coconut oil
2 boneless, skinless chicken breasts
   Salt and pepper to taste
1 clove garlic, minced
1 small onion, thinly sliced
1/2 red pepper, sliced
1/2 green or yellow pepper, sliced
1 cup zucchini, diced
1/4 cup green olives, pitted and halved
1/2 pint cherry tomatoes
   Fresh lime juice
1/8 cup chopped fresh cilantro
1/4 avocado, sliced

Heat the oil in a large skillet over medium heat. Place the chicken in the pan, season with salt and pepper and cook until no longer pink and lightly browned, about 10 to 15 minutes. Transfer the chicken to a plate and cover with aluminum foil.

Add the garlic, onions, peppers and zucchini to the skillet and cook until soft. Then add the olives and tomatoes. Cook until the tomatoes are soft, approximately 2 minutes. Remove from the heat and add the lime juice and cilantro. Serve over the chicken breasts garnished with the sliced avocado.

Calories 255 | Protein 31 g | Fat 10 g | Carbohydrates 13 g | Fiber 4 g

Protein-topped Feta and Peach Salad (Serves 2)

 1 tablespoon extra-virgin olive oil
2–3 tablespoons apple cider vinegar
     Salt and pepper to taste
 1 small package (about 4 cups) baby arugula, washed and dried
 1/4 Spanish onion, sliced
 2 ounces goat's or sheep's-milk feta
 2 large peaches, sliced (substitute: 2 cups watermelon, cubed, rind removed)

Mix the oil, vinegar, salt and pepper in a bowl. Combine the arugula and onion in another larger bowl. Add your desired amount of dressing. Top with the goat cheese and fruit, gently toss and enjoy with your choice of protein: 2 large grilled shrimp, 4 ounces grilled chicken, 3 hard-boiled egg whites or 4 ounces sliced roasted turkey per person.
Calories 298 | Protein 23 g | Fat 15 g | Carbohydrates 21 g | Fiber 4 g

Goat Cheese, Pear and Pine Nut Spinach Salad (Serves 2)

 2 tablespoons fresh lemon juice
 1 tablespoon extra-virgin olive oil
     Salt and pepper to taste
 1 package baby spinach, washed and dried
 2 tablespoons toasted pine nuts
 1 pear, thinly sliced
 1 tablespoon goat cheese, soft

In a small bowl, mix the lemon juice and olive oil. Season with salt and pepper to taste. On 2 separate plates, divide the baby spinach, pine nuts, pear slices and goat cheese. Drizzle with the dressing and top with your choice of protein: 3 large grilled shrimp, 5 ounces grilled chicken, 4 hard-boiled egg whites or 5 ounces sliced roasted turkey per person.
Calories 266 | Protein 21 g | Fat 13 g | Carbohydrates 19 g | Fiber 5 g

Roasted Beet, Orange, Walnut and Baby Arugula Salad (Serves 2)

- 1 large red or yellow beet (or 1 small red and 1 small yellow beet)
- 1 navel orange
- 1 tablespoon apple cider vinegar
- 1 tablespoon extra-virgin olive oil
- 1 teaspoon Dijon mustard or $1/2$ teaspoon dry mustard powder
  Salt and pepper to taste
- 1 package baby arugula (about 4 cups), washed and dried
- 1 ounce goat cheese, soft
- 3–4 chopped walnuts

Preheat the oven to 450°F. Wrap the beet(s) in foil and bake until tender when poked with a fork (approximately 45 to 50 minutes). Once cooled, peel the beets (wear gloves or use paper towel to avoid staining your hands) and slice into wedges.

While the beets are baking, prepare the orange by cutting off the ends of the fruit and peeling away the rind and white pith. Over a bowl, slice between the membranes and remove the whole segments. Place the segments in a separate bowl, reserving the juice to add to the dressing.

Mix the vinegar, oil, mustard and orange juice in a bowl. Add salt and pepper to taste. Toss with the arugula. Divide the arugula between 2 plates, topping with half of the beets, goat cheese, orange wedges and walnuts.

Top with your choice of protein: 2 to 3 large grilled shrimp, 4 ounces grilled chicken, 4 hard-boiled egg whites or 4 ounces sliced roasted turkey per person.

Calories 312 | Protein 29 g | Fat 15 g | Carbohydrates 16 g | Fiber 4 g

Easy Egg, Cheese and Spinach Salad (Serves 2)

- ¹/₂ large package (about 6 cups) baby spinach, washed and dried
- 2 1-inch cubes of Cabot 75% less fat Cheddar or reduced fat Swiss or Jarlsberg, grated or crumbled
- 2 hard-boiled large eggs, peeled and chopped
- 2 hard-boiled egg whites, chopped
- 1 apple, sliced
- 1 shallot, minced

In a large bowl mix the spinach, cheese, chopped egg, apple slices and minced shallot. Top with 1 to 2 tablespoons of Vinaigrette Dressing (below). Divide between 2 plates.

Calories 269 | Protein 23 g | Fat 13 g | Carbohydrates 15 g | Fiber 3 g

Vinaigrette Dressing (Serves 6)

- 1–2 tablespoons apple cider vinegar (or balsamic)
- ¹/₄ cup extra-virgin olive oil
- ¹/₂–1 teaspoon mustard powder
- Maple syrup or honey to taste
- Sea salt and pepper to taste

Mix apple cider vinegar or balsamic vinegar with the extra-virgin olive oil in a glass jar. Add mustard powder and shake to mix. Add the maple syrup or honey to your desired sweetness—keep in mind that less is more! Add sea salt and pepper to taste. This homemade dressing is great to have on hand and will keep in the fridge.

Calories 85 | Protein 0 g | Fat 9 g | Carbohydrates 0 g | Fiber 0 g

Puréed Squash and Apple Soup (Serves 4)

- 2 tablespoons extra-virgin olive oil
- 1 small onion, finely chopped
- 1 Granny Smith apple, cored, peeled and finely chopped
- 1 cup unsweetened apple cider
- 1 teaspoon ground ginger
- 1 teaspoon ground cinnamon
- 3 1/2 cups organic low-sodium vegetable stock
- 3 12-ounce packages frozen squash purée (You can make your own purée by baking 3 acorn squashes, halved and seeded, at 400°F until soft. When cool enough to touch, spoon the flesh into a food processor. Process until smooth.)
- Salt and pepper to taste

In a large pot, heat the oil and cook the onion until soft and lightly browned. Add the apples and cider and cook until the apples soften. Add the ginger, cinnamon and vegetable stock and bring to a boil. Stir in the squash purée and cook until heated through, about 8 to 10 minutes. Reduce heat and simmer until thickened. Use a hand blender to purée the mixture. Season with salt and pepper.

Ladle into 4 bowls and serve each topped with 1/4 cup crumbled pressed organic cottage cheese, 2 tablespoons plain Fage total classic yogurt or 2 1-inch cubes of crumbled Cabot 75% less fat Cheddar or reduced fat Swiss or Jarlsberg as a source of protein.

This soup may be kept in the fridge for 3 days or frozen in an airtight glass container for up to 1 month.

Calories 357 | Protein 28 g | Fat 12 g | Carbohydrates 31 g | Fiber 3 g

Japanese Spinach Salad (Serves 1)

2–3 cups fresh spinach

$1/2$ large carrot, grated

1–2 cups diced cucumber

1 small apple, grated

Rice Wine Vinegar Dressing:

2 teaspoons extra-virgin olive oil

1 teaspoon rice wine vinegar

$1/2$ teaspoon fresh grated ginger

Toss the spinach with the carrot, cucumber and apple. Mix the dressing ingredients together and drizzle over the salad. If not using this as a vegetable side dish, top with your choice of protein: 2 large grilled shrimp, 4 ounces grilled chicken, 3 hard-boiled egg whites or 4 ounces sliced roasted turkey.

Calories 358 | Protein 34 g | Fat 14 g | Carbohydrates 32 g | Fiber 7 g

Summer Raspberry Salad (Serves 1)

2 cups baby spinach leaves

1 cup chopped romaine lettuce

1 cup sugar snap peas

$1/2$ pint fresh raspberries, picked over, washed and gently dried

1 ounce goat cheese, crumbled

1 green onion, thinly sliced

1 (3 ounce) boneless, skinless chicken breast, grilled and sliced

1 recipe Rice Wine Vinegar Dressing (above)

Toss the spinach and romaine together in a bowl. Toss remaining ingredients with 1 to 2 tablespoons of the Rice Wine Vinegar Dressing (above). Top with grilled chicken breast.

Calories 345 | Protein 32 g | Fat 13 g | Carbohydrates 29 g | Fiber 12 g

Low-Fat Caesar Salad with Grilled Chicken or Shrimp (Serves 1)

Dressing:

- 1 teaspoon Dijon mustard
- 2 tablespoons fresh lemon juice
- 1 teaspoon white wine vinegar
- 1 clove garlic, crushed
   Salt and pepper to taste
- 1 teaspoon extra-virgin olive oil
- 1 tablespoon chia seeds
- $^1/_3$ cup plain nonfat yogurt or goat milk yogurt
- 1 teaspoon Worcestershire sauce

Place the mustard, lemon juice, vinegar, garlic and salt and pepper in a small food processor and mix until well blended. Add the olive oil, chia seeds, yogurt and Worcestershire sauce and process again until creamy. Taste and adjust seasoning with salt and pepper. Use 1 to 2 tablespoons of the dressing per salad. The remainder can be kept in an airtight container in the fridge for 3 to 4 days.

Salad:

- 3 cups romaine lettuce
- 2 teaspoons grated Parmesan (optional)

Toss the romaine, dressing and Parmesan together in a bowl. Top your salad with 2 large grilled shrimp or 3 ounces grilled chicken breast.

Calories 282 | Protein 29 g | Fat 14 g | Carbohydrates 17 g | Fiber 7 g

Roasted Vegetable Soup (Serves 4)

- 6 beefsteak tomatoes, halved and cored
- 2 carrots, in 1/2-inch slices
- 1 small zucchini, in 1/2-inch slices
- 1 large onion, sliced
- 1 sweet potato, in 1/2-inch slices (omit this if making the soup in week 1)
- 2 leeks, white and light green parts only, thoroughly washed and cut into 1/2-inch pieces
- 1 teaspoon dried thyme
- 4–5 cloves garlic
- 2 tablespoons extra-virgin olive oil
- Salt and pepper to taste
- 4 cups organic low-sodium vegetable broth (such as Imagine Organic Low-Sodium Vegetable Broth)

Preheat the oven to 425°F. Place the tomatoes (cut side down), carrots, zucchini, onion, sweet potato, leeks, thyme and garlic in a single layer on a large roasting pan. Drizzle with the olive oil and season with salt and pepper. Roast until tender, approximately 45 to 60 minutes. Once the vegetables are cooled, peel the tomatoes, discarding the skins, and transfer the vegetables to a large pot on the stove top. Add the vegetable broth (add more broth or water if needed). Bring to a boil then reduce and simmer for 10 to 20 minutes. Use a hand blender to purée the mixture until smooth. Ladle into 4 bowls and serve each topped with 1/4 cup crumbled pressed organic cottage cheese, 2 to 3 tablespoons plain Fage total 0% Greek yogurt or 2 1-inch cubes of crumbled Cabot 75% less fat Cheddar as a source of protein.

This soup can be kept in the fridge for up to 3 days.

Calories 282 | Protein 26 g | Fat 10 g | Carbohydrates 22 g | Fiber 5 g

Tasty Toasted Tuna Salad (Serves 2)

- $^1/_2$ cup chopped celery
- 1 small onion, chopped
- $^1/_2$ cup low-fat cottage cheese
- 1 can (6 ounces) Raincoast Tuna, drained and flaked
- 1 $^1/_2$ tablespoons low-fat or olive oil–based Hellmann's mayonnaise
- 1 tablespoon lemon juice
- 1 Ezekiel English muffin, halved

Preheat the oven to 350°F. In a large skillet over low heat, cook the celery and onion until softened. Add the cottage cheese, tuna, mayo and lemon juice to the skillet. Continue to cook the mixture until the cheese melts and the mixture is warmed through.

Divide the mixture between the English muffin halves. Place the muffin halves on a baking sheet, and bake for 10 minutes.

Calories 292 | Protein 28 g | Fat 10 g | Carbohydrates 24 g | Fiber 5 g

Tasty Toasted Tuna Salad

Brie's Fresh and Easy Baby Spinach Salad (Serves 2)

- 6 cups baby spinach
- $^1/_2$ cup fresh raspberries
- $^1/_2$ cup fresh blueberries
- 1 small apple, chopped
- $^1/_4$ cup crumbled feta cheese
- 6 ounces skinless, boneless chicken breast, grilled and sliced
- 2 teaspoons low-sugar, canola- or olive oil–based salad dressing

Mix the spinach, berries, apple and feta in a bowl. Toss with the dressing. Divide the salad between 2 plates and top with the grilled chicken.

Calories 277 | Protein 25 g | Fat 12 g | Carbohydrates 22 g | Fiber 6 g

Brie's Fresh and Easy Baby Spinach Salad

Dinner Recipes

Rice Pasta with Chicken, Goat Cheese and Roasted Asparagus (Serves 4)

- 4 small boneless, skinless chicken breasts (approximately 4 ounces each)
- 2 bunches young asparagus
- 1 tablespoon extra-virgin olive oil
- 1 tablespoon unsalted butter
  Juice of half a fresh lemon, plus lemon slices
  Salt and pepper to taste
- 1 cup dried rice pasta (spiral or another short pasta shape)
- 3 ounces goat cheese
- 2 tablespoons chopped fresh chives

Preheat the oven to 450°F. Place the chicken on one roasting pan and the asparagus on another. Drizzle the asparagus with the olive oil, dot with 1 tablespoon of the butter and season with the lemon juice and salt and pepper. Place lemon slices on the chicken and season with chives, salt and pepper. Put the chicken in the oven first. Ten minutes later, put the asparagus in the oven. Bake both for another 15 minutes, or until the asparagus is tender and the chicken is cooked through. Cut the asparagus and chicken into 1- to 2-inch pieces.

In the meantime, boil the rice pasta until al dente. Reserving 1 cup of the pasta water, drain the pasta and return to the pot.

In another bowl, combine the cheese and 1/2 cup of the hot pasta water. Season with salt and pepper and whisk until smooth.

Add the goat cheese mixture, chicken and the asparagus to the pasta pot. Toss with the pasta. If there is not enough cheese mixture to cover all of the noodles, add more pasta water to the pot.

Calories 338 | Protein 33 g | Fat 13 g | Carbohydrates 25 g | Fiber 3 g

Kamut Pasta with Peas and Ricotta (Serves 4)

- 1 cup dried kamut or buckwheat penne, fusilli or spaghetti (or another gluten-free pasta)
- $1/2$ package frozen spinach (defrosted and drained)
- 1 cup frozen baby peas
- 1 tablespoon unsalted butter
- 1 clove garlic, minced
- 1 tablespoon olive oil
- 2 $1/2$ cups low-fat ricotta cheese
- 2–3 fresh basil leaves, chopped
  Sea salt and pepper to taste

Bring a pot of water to a boil with generous amounts of sea salt added. Add the pasta and cook until al dente. In the last few minutes of cooking, add the spinach and frozen peas to the boiling pasta. Reserving $1/2$ cup of pasta water, drain the pasta and peas. Return the pasta and peas to the pot.

Toss the pasta and peas with the butter, olive oil, garlic, ricotta cheese and half the chopped basil. Add the pasta water to create a thin sauce that coats the pasta. Season with salt and pepper. Serve in pasta bowls and garnish with the remaining fresh basil.

Calories 320 | Protein 26 g | Fat 10 g | Carbohydrates 34 g | Fiber 7 g

Whole Roasted Chicken and Herb-baked Sweet Potato Fries (Serves 4)

Roasted Chicken:

1	roasting chicken, about 4–5 pounds
	Juice of $\frac{1}{2}$ lemon
	Salt and pepper to taste
1	small onion, quartered
$\frac{1}{4}$	teaspoon dried rosemary
$\frac{1}{2}$	teaspoon dried thyme
2–3	tablespoons roughly chopped fresh parsley
1	tablespoon melted butter

Preheat the oven to 350°F. Rub the cavity of the chicken with lemon juice; sprinkle with salt and pepper. Place the onion quarters, rosemary, thyme and parsley in the chicken cavity. Place the chicken in a shallow roasting pan and roast for about 20 minutes per pound. Baste with the melted butter halfway through baking. The internal temperature should register about 165°F on a meat thermometer inserted into the meaty part of the thigh.

Serve the chicken (about 4 to 5 ounces per person) with the fries and a side salad of mixed greens.

Sweet Potato Fries:

	Non-stick olive oil spray
1	pound sweet potatoes, peeled, cut into $\frac{1}{2}$-inch batons
1–2	tablespoons extra-virgin olive oil
	Salt and pepper to taste
	Herbamare Spicy Aromatic Sea Salt to taste (optional)
2	tablespoons chopped fresh Italian parsley
1	teaspoon chopped fresh thyme or $\frac{1}{2}$ teaspoon dried
1	clove garlic, minced

Spray a large baking sheet with olive oil spray. In a large bowl, toss the sweet potatoes with the olive oil. Sprinkle generously with salt and pepper. Spread the sweet potatoes in a single layer on the prepared baking sheet. If desired, sprinkle with seasoned sea salt.

Place the fries in the oven about 30 to 40 minutes before the chicken is done. Bake until the sweet potatoes are tender and golden brown, turning once at about 15 minutes.

Mix the parsley, thyme and garlic in a small bowl. Remove the sweet potatoes from oven and toss with the parsley mixture before serving.

Calories 369 | Protein 30 g | Fat 13 g | Carbohydrates 33 g | Fiber 5 g

Tomato Turkey Delight (Serves 2)

2	tablespoons extra-virgin olive oil
1	cup onions, chopped
1–2	cloves garlic, crushed
8	ounces ground turkey
1 1/2	cups crushed tomatoes
1/2–1	teaspoon chili powder or chipotle spice
1	cup zucchini, chopped
3	cups frozen or fresh green beans
	Salt and pepper to taste

Heat the oil in a large skillet and cook the onion, garlic and ground turkey until meat is completely cooked (no longer pink), and the onions are soft. Add the tomato, chili powder or chipotle spice and the zucchini and cook until heated through. In the meantime, steam the green beans. Divide the cooked beans between 2 plates and top with the turkey mixture.

Calories 313 | Protein 27 g | Fat 12 g | Carbohydrates 28 g | Fiber 9 g

Carb-conscious Lasagna (Serves 10)

- 2 pounds ground turkey
- 1 clove garlic, minced
  Salt and pepper to taste
- 1 (8-ounce) can tomato sauce
- 1 teaspoon Italian seasoning
- 2 whole omega-3 eggs
- 15 ounces low-fat ricotta cheese
  Pinch chopped parsley
- 3/4 cup low-fat shredded mozzarella cheese
- 2–3 whole zucchinis
- 1/4 cup grated Parmesan cheese

Preheat oven to 325°F. In a skillet, cook the turkey with the garlic and season with salt and pepper. When the turkey is fully cooked, drain excess water and then stir in the tomato sauce and Italian seasoning.

In a separate dish, beat the eggs with the ricotta; add a little salt and pepper and the parsley. Set aside.

Thinly slice the unpeeled zucchinis lengthwise about 1/8 inch thick. Grease a 9- × 13-inch baking pan and layer the ingredients in the pan: one-third of the zucchini, salt and pepper; half the meat sauce, one-third of the zucchini, salt and pepper; all of the ricotta, half the mozzarella and Parmesan, one-third of the zucchini, salt and pepper; the rest of the meat sauce; the rest of the cheeses. Bake at 325°F for 45 to 60 minutes until bubbly and the zucchini is cooked well. Can be frozen. Enjoy with grilled vegetables or 1/2 cup cooked quinoa.

Calories 356 | Protein 34 g | Fat 13 g | Carbohydrates 25 g | Fiber 4 g

Tilapia with Fresh Tropical Salsa (Serves 2)

Salsa:

- 2   Roma tomatoes, diced
- 1/4 cup diced fresh mango or pineapple
- 1   tablespoon diced red onion
- 1   tablespoon lime juice
-     Splash extra-virgin olive oil
-     Finely chopped fresh cilantro
-     Salt and pepper to taste

Mix together all ingredients in a bowl.

Tilapia:

- 2   tilapia fillets
-     Splash of extra-virgin olive oil
- 1/4 teaspoon dried rosemary, thyme or dill (your preference)
-     Lemon slices
-     Salt and pepper to taste
- 1   acorn squash, washed, halved and seeds removed

Preheat the oven to 425°F. Place squash in a baking dish, flesh side up. Drizzle with olive oil and season with salt and pepper. Bake until soft, about 45 minutes. Place the tilapia in a baking dish and add the olive oil, herbs and lemon slices to fillets. Bake for 15 minutes. Serve the fresh salsa over the baked tilapia and half a medium-size baked acorn squash per person. Season with salt and pepper.

Calories 315 | Protein 24 g | Fat 11 g | Carbohydrates 30 g | Fiber 5 g

Curried Ginger Chicken Breast with Quinoa (Serves 2)

Chicken:

   2   green onions, minced
   $^1/_2$ tablespoon fresh ginger, peeled and finely grated
   1   teaspoon curry powder
   1   tablespoon fresh lime juice
       Salt and pepper to taste
   2   (4–5 ounces) bone-in, skinless chicken breasts

Preheat the oven to 375°F. In a small bowl, combine the green onions, ginger, curry powder, lime juice and salt and pepper. Place the chicken in a baking dish and cover each piece with the seasoning mixture. Bake until cooked through, turning once, about 20 to 25 minutes.

Meanwhile, prepare the side dish:

Quinoa:

   1   cup water
   1   cup quinoa, rinsed
   1   cup frozen baby peas
       Salt and pepper to taste
   $^1/_4$ cup cilantro, chopped
   2   teaspoons extra-virgin olive oil

In a small saucepan, bring the water to a boil. Add the quinoa, baby peas and salt. Bring to a boil. Reduce heat to low, cover and simmer until the quinoa is tender and has absorbed all the liquid, 11 to 13 minutes. Remove from the heat and toss in the cilantro and olive oil. Season with salt and pepper and serve as a side dish with the chicken.

Calories 328 | Protein 31 g | Fat 10 g | Carbohydrates 30 g | Fiber 6 g

Chicken Stir-fry with Peppers and Fresh Basil (Serves 2)

2	tablespoons coconut oil
2	boneless, skinless chicken breasts, sliced
1	small onion, sliced
1	red pepper, sliced
1	green pepper, sliced
2–3	cloves garlic, minced
$^1/_4$–$^1/_3$	cup water
2	tablespoons tamari sauce
1	tablespoon rice wine vinegar
$^3/_4$	cup Thai basil leaves
1	tablespoon chopped lemongrass

Heat half the oil in a skillet and cook the chicken until almost done, about 3 minutes. Put the chicken aside. Wipe the pan with a paper towel and add the remaining oil to the skillet. Heat over medium heat, then add the onion and peppers. Cook until soft and beginning to brown, about 3 to 4 minutes. Add the garlic and cook for 1 more minute.

Add the water, tamari, vinegar and chicken to the pan. Cook, tossing until the chicken is thoroughly cooked. Remove from the heat, fold in the basil leaves and chopped lemongrass and serve over $^1/_4$ cup cooked basmati rice.

Calories 300 | Protein 29 g | Fat 10 g | Carbohydrates 25 g | Fiber 3 g

Mediterranean Chicken Kebabs with Greek Dipping Sauce (Serves 2)

2   boneless, skinless chicken breasts, cut into 1-inch pieces
1   red pepper, diced
1   red onion, quartered, root removed and layers separated
1   zucchini, halved then cut into 1-inch slices
2   teaspoons extra-virgin olive oil
$^1/_2$ teaspoon oregano
2   tablespoons balsamic vinegar
    Salt and pepper to taste
    Wooden or metal skewers

In a resealable bag or large glass bowl, combine the chicken, red pepper, red onion, zucchini, olive oil, oregano and balsamic vinegar; season with salt and pepper. Marinate for 30 to 40 minutes or refrigerate overnight.

If using wooden skewers, soak them in cold water for about 30 minutes before assembling your kebabs.

Prepare the barbecue or grill by lightly brushing oil on the rack to prevent sticking. Prepare the skewers by dividing the zucchini, chicken, onion and peppers among 4 skewers. Grill the skewers, turning frequently, until the chicken is cooked through and the vegetables are tender, about 13 to 15 minutes.

Dipping Sauce:

$^1/_4$ cup crumbled feta
$^1/_4$ cup plain goat milk yogurt
1   tablespoon fresh dill
$^1/_2$ cup fresh mint leaves

To make the dipping sauce, place the feta, yogurt, dill and fresh mint in a food processor. Blend until smooth. Season with salt and pepper. Serve with the kebabs.

Option: Serve with side of $^1/_4$ cup cooked basmati rice.

Calories 373 | Protein 33 g | Fat 14 g | Carbohydrates 31 g | Fiber 4 g

Almond-crusted Chicken Breasts with Herbed New Potatoes and Baby Arugula Salad (Serves 2)

Potatoes:

- ³/₄ pound new red potatoes (this provides each person with ¹/₂ to ³/₄ cup potatoes)
- ¹/₂ tablespoon extra-virgin olive oil
  Mixed herbs including oregano, thyme, rosemary, etc.
  Herbamare Aromatic Sea Salt and pepper to taste

Preheat the oven to 450°F. Toss the potatoes with the olive oil and herbs. Season with salt and pepper. Place in a single layer in a pan for roasting. Cook, turning once or twice, until golden brown, about 30 to 40 minutes.

Meanwhile prepare the chicken:

Almond-crusted Chicken Breasts:

- ¹/₄ cup ground almonds (or almond flour)
  Salt and pepper
- 2 skinless, boneless chicken breasts
- 2 egg whites, beaten

Mix the ground almonds with salt and pepper. Dip the chicken into the egg whites then into the almond mixture. Completely coat the chicken and place on a baking sheet. After the potatoes have been roasting for about 20 to 25 minutes, put the chicken into the hot oven. Cook, without turning, 10 to 15 minutes, until cooked through.

When the chicken is almost done, prepare the arugula:

Baby Arugula Salad:

- 1 small Spanish onion, thinly sliced
- 1–2 tablespoons fresh lemon juice
- 1 teaspoon extra-virgin olive oil
  Salt and pepper to taste
- 3–4 cups baby arugula

Toss the onion, lemon juice, olive oil and salt and pepper in a bowl. Add the arugula and toss to coat. Remove the chicken and potatoes from the oven. Serve with the salad.

Calories 337 | Protein 34 g | Fat 13 g | Carbohydrates 22 g | Fiber 4 g

Coconut Chicken Curry with Rice (Serves 2)

1	tablespoon coconut oil
2	skinless, boneless chicken breasts, sliced
1	tablespoon fresh lime juice
1	red onion, sliced
1	red pepper, sliced
2	heads baby bok choy, sliced lengthwise
2–3	tablespoons water
$^1/_2$–1	tablespoon red curry paste (check that it is free of harmful oils)
$^1/_2$–$^3/_4$	can low-fat, unsweetened coconut milk
$^1/_2$	cup fresh basil leaves
	Salt and pepper to taste
Optional:	$^1/_2$ cup cooked rice noodles (vermicelli) or $^1/_2$ cup cooked basmati rice

Heat the oil in a large skillet over medium heat. Add the chicken to the pan and cook until browned and almost cooked through. Add the fresh lime juice. Transfer to a plate and keep warm.

Add the red onion, red pepper, bok choy and water to the pan and cook until the vegetables are tender-crisp, about 4 minutes. Add the curry paste and cook 1 to 2 minutes more, stirring. Add the chicken and the coconut milk and stir to combine. Simmer until the sauce thickens, about 8 to 10 minutes. Remove from heat and add the basil. Season with salt and pepper and serve over rice noodles or cooked basmati rice if desired.

Calories 356 | Protein 29 g | Fat 12 g | Carbohydrates 33 g | Fiber 3 g

Curried Shrimp (Serves 2)

- 1 tablespoon coconut or extra-virgin olive oil
- 1 small onion, thinly sliced
- Salt to taste
- 1 tablespoon tomato paste
- $1/2$–$1/4$ teaspoon ground ginger
- 1 teaspoon curry powder
- 2 Roma tomatoes, quartered and cut into large chunks
- $3/4$ cup water
- $1/2$ pound fresh or frozen shrimp, peeled and uncooked
- 3–4 tablespoons low-fat yogurt, plain
- Fresh lime juice
- $1/2$ cup cooked basmati rice or jasmine rice

Heat the oil in a skillet over medium heat. Add the onion, season with salt and cook until softened. Add the tomato paste, ginger and curry. Cook for another minute or so, stirring until the curry is fully dispersed.

Add the tomatoes and cook until they release their juices, about 1 minute. Add the water and simmer another 3 to 5 minutes. Add the shrimp and cook until opaque, about 4 minutes. Remove from the heat.

Add the yogurt and fresh lime juice to taste. Serve over the rice.

Calories 328 | Protein 32 g | Fat 9 g | Carbohydrates 29 g | Fiber 4 g

Sweet Potato Pancakes (Serves 2; 2 pancakes each)

2   medium-size sweet potatoes, peeled and coarsely grated or
     shredded in a food processor
2   green onions, finely chopped
     Salt and pepper to taste
5   egg whites, beaten
¹/₄ cup almond flour
¹/₂ teaspoon paprika
2–3 tablespoons extra-virgin olive oil or coconut oil

In a large bowl, mix the sweet potatoes, green onions, salt and pepper, egg whites, flour and paprika. Use one quarter of the mixture to form each pancake, 4 in total. In a skillet over medium heat, cook each in the oil until golden brown. (As a low-fat option, you can bake the pancakes on an oiled baking sheet.) Serve hot with a healthy dose of protein such as 2 to 3 ounces of grilled chicken or turkey breast.

Calories 260 | Protein 14 g | Fat 12 g | Carbohydrates 27 g | Fiber 5 g

Refreshing Cucumber and Dill Salad (Serves 2)

¹/₄ cup plain yogurt or goat yogurt
1   tablespoon fresh lemon juice
1   tablespoon chopped fresh dill
2   teaspoons chopped fresh chives
1   tablespoon extra-vrigin olive oil
1   English cucumber, cut in half lengthwise and thinly sliced
     Salt and pepper to taste

Whisk the yogurt, lemon juice, dill, chives, olive oil and salt and pepper in a small bowl. Add to the cucumber; toss until the cucumber is completely coated with the mixture. Serve.

Calories 94 | Protein 2 g | Fat 7 g | Carbohydrates 8 g | Fiber 1 g

Roasted Chicken Breasts (Serves 2)

- 2 boneless, skinless chicken breasts
- 10 asparagus spears, trimmed
- 2 Roma tomatoes, diced
- 1 tablespoon extra-virgin olive oil
- 1/4 teaspoon dried rosemary
- 1/4 teaspoon dried thyme
- 1/4 cup low-sodium chicken stock
     Salt and pepper to taste

Preheat the oven to 400°F. Place the chicken, asparagus and tomatoes in a medium-size baking or casserole dish and drizzle the olive oil over top. Season well with salt and pepper, rosemary and thyme. Pour the chicken stock over the chicken and cover with foil. Bake for 25 to 35 minutes. Enjoy with a side salad or baked squash.

Calories 230 | Protein 28 g | Fat 11 g | Carbohydrates 9 g | Fiber 4 g

Pecan-crusted Chicken Breasts with Steamed Asparagus and Rapini (Serves 4)

- 2 acorn squash, washed, quartered and seeds removed
- 10–15 Mary's Crackers
- 3/4 cup pecans
- 1 tablespoon extra-virgin olive oil plus more for the baking sheet
  Salt and pepper to taste
- 1/4 cup egg whites
- 4 boneless, skinless chicken breasts (approximately 4 ounces each)
- 1 bunch rapini, chopped
- 1 bunch young asparagus
- 1 tablespoon extra-virgin olive oil
- 2 teaspoons finely grated lemon zest

Preheat the oven to 475°F. Place squash in a baking dish, flesh side up. Drizzle with olive oil and season with salt and pepper. Bake until soft, about 30 minutes.

Place the Mary's Crackers, pecans and olive oil in a food processor and pulse until coarsely ground. Add 1 teaspoon salt and 1/4 teaspoon pepper. Pour this mixture onto a large plate.

In another bowl, lightly whisk the egg whites, then season generously with salt and pepper. Dip the chicken into the egg mixture, making sure to coat all sides. Next, dip the chicken into the pecan and cracker mixture, coating completely. Place the chicken on a baking sheet and bake until cooked through, about 15 minutes.

While the chicken is baking, put a small amount of water in the bottom of a steamer. Place the rapini and asparagus in the top of the steamer. When they are tender crisp, transfer to a bowl and toss with the olive oil and lemon zest. Season with salt and pepper to taste. Serve the chicken breasts with the rapini and asparagus and baked squash.

Calories 354 | Protein 34 g | Fat 14 g | Carbohydrates 31 g | Fiber 5 g

Perfect Pesto Chicken with Cauliflower Mash (Serves 2)
Pesto Chicken:
- 2   tablespoons fresh basil leaves
- 1   tablespoon extra-virgin olive oil or macadamia nut oil
- 1   tablespoon pine nuts or slivered almonds
- 1   tablespoon grated Parmesan cheese
- 2   boneless, skinless chicken breasts (approximately 4–5 ounces each)

Preheat the oven to 350°F. Place the basil, oil, nuts and Parmesan in a food processor and blend until well mixed. Spread the pesto mixture over each chicken breast and bake until cooked through, about 20 to 25 minutes.

Note: You can purchase a prepared pesto product, but ensure the product you purchase contains only olive oil, no sugar.

Cauliflower Mash:
- 1/2   small yellow onion, diced (optional)
- 1   large head cauliflower
     Kosher salt
- 2   cloves garlic, minced (or 2 tablespoons roasted garlic)
     Freshly ground pepper

Bring a large pot of water to a boil. In another pot, carefully sauté the onion until lightly browned. (The onions are optional, but they add flavor).

Remove any green leaves then cut the head of cauliflower into large chunks. Include the stems, but discard the main core. Add several dashes of kosher salt to the boiling water and then add the cauliflower. Lower the heat and cook until the cauliflower is fork-tender, about 15 minutes. Reserving a cup of the boiling water, drain the cauliflower.

Add the garlic to the onions and cook till soft (if using roasted garlic, add directly to the drained cauliflower). Transfer the onion and garlic mixture to a food processor and purée to a smooth paste, adding a splash of the water from the cauliflower if needed.

Drain the cauliflower and either mash with a fork for a chunky texture or place in the food processor for a smoother consistency. Do not overprocess, or the cauliflower will become gummy. Fold in the onion-garlic paste and add salt and pepper to taste.

Calories 321 | Protein 32 g | Fat 13 g | Carbohydrates 19 g | Fiber 9 g

Grilled Veggie and Sea Scallop Kebabs (Serves 2)

1¹/₂ tablespoon extra-virgin olive oil
  1 tablespoon lemon juice
  1 teaspoon fresh thyme
    Salt and pepper to taste
 10 ounces sea scallops or as many as you need for 4–6 skewers
  4 shallots, halved
  1 green pepper, diced
  1 red pepper, diced
  1 small zucchini, sliced into ³/₄-inch rounds
  6 cherry tomatoes
    Wooden or metal skewers

Combine 1 tablespoon of the olive oil with the lemon juice, thyme and salt and pepper. Rub this mixture into the scallops. Cover and marinate for about 15 to 20 minutes.

If using wooden skewers, soak them in cold water for about 30 minutes before assembling your kebabs.

Preheat the grill to medium-high (if you don't have a grill you can do this under the broiler on a pan). Prepare the barbecue or grill.

Alternate scallops with chunks of vegetables on the skewers. Brush the kebabs with the remaining olive oil and season generously with salt and pepper. Grill for 2 to 3 minutes per side. Let them rest and serve on a bed of baby greens. Enjoy with side salad or cooked quinoa (week 2 only).

Calories 304 | Protein 31 g | Fat 12 g | Carbohydrates 21 g | Fiber 7 g

Baked Halibut Topped with Broiled Tomato-Mango Salsa (Serves 2)

Broiled Tomato-Mango Salsa:

- 1 pound very ripe Roma tomatoes
- 1 ripe mango
- 1 teaspoon chopped cilantro
- 1 tablespoon extra-virgin olive oil
- 1/4 cup fresh lime juice
  Salt and freshly ground pepper to taste

Preheat the broiler. Halve the tomatoes and transfer to a shallow baking pan, cut side up. Broil the tomatoes until slightly charred, about 15 minutes. Remove from the heat and set aside.

Peel mango. Roughly chop tomatoes, mango and cilantro and mix with olive oil and lime juice in a bowl. Add salt and pepper to taste.

Baked Halibut:

- 2 fillets (4–5 ounces each) fresh halibut
- 1/2 tablespoon extra-virgin olive oil

Preheat the oven to 350°F while the tomatoes are cooling. Arrange the fish fillets in a shallow baking dish, drizzled with the oil and bake until tender, approximately 15 minutes. When the fish is done, top with the salsa and serve.

Calories 326 | Protein 27 g | Fat 14 g | Carbohydrates 29 g | Fiber 6 g

Chicken Chili (Serves 8)

- 1 tablespoon extra-virgin olive oil
- 2 tablespoons finely chopped fresh ginger
- 6 green onions, chopped
- 4 cloves garlic, finely chopped
- 2 sweet red peppers, diced
- 1 orange pepper, diced
- 2 teaspoons chili paste (optional)
- 1 pound boneless, skinless chicken breast, diced
- 1 28-ounce can organic plum tomatoes, drained and puréed
- 2 cups cooked red kidney beans or 1 (19 oz) can, rinsed and drained
- 2 cups cooked black beans or 1 (19 oz) can, rinsed and drained
- 2 tablespoons tamari sauce
- 1 tablespoon rice wine
- 1/2 cup chopped parsley (optional)

Heat the oil in a large skillet or wok on medium heat. Add the ginger, green onions and garlic and cook, stirring, for 30 seconds. Add the red and orange peppers and chili paste and cook for a few minutes, until the peppers start to soften. Add the chicken to the skillet. Cook, stirring constantly, for about 5 minutes, or until the chicken pieces are white on the outside. Add the tomatoes and bring to a boil. Reduce the heat and simmer gently for 25 minutes. Stir in the beans, tamari sauce and rice wine. Cook for 15 minutes. Stir in the parsley and enjoy.

Calories 300 | Protein 27 g | Fat 10 g | Carbohydrates 29 g | Fiber 6 g

Halibut with Roasted Tomatoes (Serves 2)

- 3 Roma tomatoes, diced
- 1 onion, diced
- 1 clove garlic, minced
- 1 tablespoon extra-virgin olive oil
  Salt and pepper to taste
- 2 halibut fillets
- $1/4$ teaspoon dried thyme
  Fresh lemon juice (optional)

Preheat the oven to 375°F. In a baking dish, mix together the tomatoes, onion and garlic. Add the oil. Season well with salt and pepper. Roast for 8 to 10 minutes until soft.

Season the halibut with salt, pepper and thyme. Spray a large skillet with non-stick spray. Over medium-high heat, sear the halibut on both sides until lightly browned.

Transfer the halibut fillets onto the roasted tomato mixture and bake for an additional 8 to 10 minutes. Squeeze the lemon juice on the halibut after it is cooked. Serve with $1/2$ cup of brown basmati rice if you are in week 2 or beyond. If in week 1, serve with baked acorn squash or side salad.

Calories 305 | Protein 28 g | Fat 10 g | Carbohydrates 28 g | Fiber 4 g

Chicken Cabbage Cashew Stir-fry (Serves 2)

2	teaspoons extra-virgin olive oil or coconut oil
8	ounces skinless chicken breast, cut into strips
¹/₄	teaspoon garlic
¹/₄	teaspoon ginger
	Salt and pepper to taste
1	small bunch broccoli florets, approximately 1 cup
¹/₂	red bell pepper, sliced
¹/₂	orange pepper, sliced
2	cups shredded cabbage
1	medium onion, sliced
1	tablespoon tamari sauce
8	cashews

Heat the oil in a large non-stick skillet or wok. Add the chicken, garlic, ginger, broccoli and peppers. Add the cabbage and onion and sauté until tender-crisp. Add the tamari sauce and cashews and cook for 1 minute. Serve on ¹/₂ cup of brown or basmati rice per person if in week 2 or beyond, or by itself if restricting grains as in week 1.

Calories 360 | Protein 32 g | Fat 14 g | Carbohydrates 32 g | Fiber 5 g

Chicken Souvlaki (Serves 2)

- 2 boneless, skinless chicken breasts
- 1 clove garlic
- 2 tablespoons lemon juice
- 2 tablespoons red wine vinegar
- $^1/_2$ teaspoon dried oregano
- $^1/_4$ teaspoon red chili flakes
- 4 teaspoons extra-virgin olive oil
  Salt and pepper
  Bamboo or metal skewers

Cut the chicken into 2-inch cubes. In a medium bowl, combine the garlic, lemon juice, vinegar, oregano, chili flakes, oil and salt and pepper. Marinate the chicken for an hour.

If using bamboo skewers, soak them in cold water for about 30 minutes before assembling your kebabs, then thread chicken onto skewers.

Preheat the grill to medium heat. Prepare the barbecue or grill by lightly brushing oil on the rack to prevent sticking. Grill the chicken until cooked through. (The marinade also works great on whole chicken breasts.) Serve with $^1/_2$ cup basmati rice (only if in week 2 or beyond).

Calories 308 | Protein 26 g | Fat 12 g | Carbohydrates 23 g | Fiber 3 g

Sauces and Dressings
Quick-and-Easy Red Pepper Sauce (Serves 3)

- 2 tablespoons extra-virgin olive oil
- 1 small red pepper, minced or diced (depending on how you like the texture of your sauce)
- $^1/_2$ small red onion, minced
- 1 teaspoon paprika
- $^1/_2$ teaspoon ground cumin
- $^1/_4$ teaspoon cayenne
- 3 cloves garlic, minced, or 1 tablespoon garlic powder
- 1 teaspoon Herbamare Spicy Aromatic Sea Salt
- $^1/_3$ cup fresh cilantro, coarsely chopped
- 2 tablespoons lemon juice
  Lemon zest

Combine the oil, pepper, onion, paprika, cumin, cayenne, garlic and salt in a saucepan. Cook on medium-high for about 5 minutes, until the vegetables are tender. Stir in the fresh cilantro, lemon juice and lemon zest immediately before serving.

*This zesty sauce is a perfect topping for grilled shrimp, chicken or any white fish. Serve over a bed of greens, with lots of fresh veggies.

Calories 178 | Protein 1 g | Fat 9 g | Carbohydrates 10 g | Fiber 2 g

Guacamole (Serves 4)

3   ripe avocados
1   Roma tomato, diced
1   tablespoon diced red onion
1   clove garlic, minced
     Hot sauce, to taste
     Chopped fresh cilantro (as desired)
     Juice of 1 lime
     Salt and pepper to taste

Mash the avocados with a fork and combine with the tomato, red onion, garlic, hot sauce, cilantro, lime juice and salt and pepper.

Serve with pita chips. Also makes a nice spread for sandwiches.

Calories 137 | Protein 1 g | Fat 13 g | Carbohydrates 3 g | Fiber 3 g

Tasty Tomato Sauce (Serves 3–4)

2   tablespoons extra-virgin olive oil
1   onion, diced
2   cloves garlic, minced
1   small zucchini, grated
1   red, yellow or orange pepper, diced
1   28-ounce can diced tomatoes
1   tablespoon tomato paste
     Bunch fresh basil, finely chopped
$1/2$ teaspoon red chili flakes
     Salt and pepper to taste

Heat the olive oil in a large skillet. Sauté onion, garlic, zucchini and pepper. Add the diced tomatoes and the tomato paste. Add the fresh basil, chili flakes and salt and pepper. Cook for 10 minutes to allow the flavors to combine.

Calories 176 | Protein 4 g | Fat 10 g | Carbohydrates 22 g | Fiber 4 g

Quick-and-Easy Balsamic Vinaigrette (Serves 12–13)

- 10 tablespoons extra-virgin olive oil
- 3 tablespoons balsamic vinegar
- 1 tablespoon lime juice
- 1/4 teaspoon Dijon mustard
- 1–2 tablespoons maple syrup or honey (or to taste)
- Salt and pepper to taste

Place all ingredients in a bottle with a lid. Shake well to combine the flavors before serving. If you make the dressing in a bowl, mix vigorously with a whisk or fork. Serve with mixed salad greens.

Calories 100 | Protein 0 g | Fat 10 g | Carbohydrates 2 g | Fiber 0 g

PART THREE

Go confidently in the direction of your dreams.
Live the life you have imagined.

HENRY DAVID THOREAU

THE HORMONE DIET
WELLNESS TRACKER

Motivation is what gets you started. Habit is what keeps you going.

JIM RYAN

Getting and staying balanced requires you to be committed, organized and motivated. To help you in all three of these areas during your *supercharged* hormonal health program, I have created the Hormone Diet Wellness Tracker. Use this tool to keep you on the road to success and optimal wellness.

Food and Drink Habits

Upon starting your *Supercharged* Hormone Diet plan, you will begin to record everything that you eat and drink daily on the Wellness Tracker sheets in the spaces allotted for each meal. The food intake checklists on the sheets match each week of the program, so that you can easily take stock of the foods you should be eating. You also need to track your water intake. Calculate the cups of water you need daily with this formula:

[Your weight] × 0.55 = number of ounces to drink daily ÷ 8 = number of cups you need daily

Hot Hormone foods are also listed. Checking off these bonus foods daily means you will have greater gains for your hormonal health. You can also keep track of any supplements you need.

During week 3 you will introduce a new food into your diet each day in an attempt to determine your food sensitivities. You'll notice that your Hot Hormone food checklist is removed during this week to provide you with a space to note and record any possible reaction you may notice from the test food. Remember to pay attention to how you feel after eating the food, as well as upon rising the next day.

Sleep Habits

Note your sleep quality, bed time and number of hours slept. Keep in mind that it's best to go to bed before 11 p.m. and to sleep at least 7.5 hours a night.

pH Balance

Record your pH each morning. Your goal is a salivary reading of 7.2 to 7.4 each morning. When it is in the normal range, you can continue to measure it only once a week when you take your weight.

Weight

I recommend that you weigh yourself at the beginning of each week only, though I know some people like to do it daily during the program. Your weight is by no means the be-all and end-all measurement of your success during this process. Remember, it's the entirety of your Best Body Assessment measurements that are most important.

Exercise Habits

Write down all of the exercise you do daily, including the type of activity, the length of your session and the intensity. Cardio and yoga are the only activities prescribed during weeks 1 to 4. Strength training three times a week is recommended at the onset of week 5.

Relaxation Habits

Pick 10 minutes per day as your time. Meditate, visualize, write your goals or just simply breathe. This could be the most important thing you do each day.

Summary of Best Body Assessments

You may wish to fill in your measurements here so that you can quickly see what you have achieved during your program, and where you still may need to go.

BEST BODY ASSESSMENT

MARKER	DAY 1	DAY 30+	GOAL/ INTERPRETATION
Weight			
Waist measurement			W < 35"; M < 40"
Hip measurement			
Waist-to-hip ratio			W < 0.80; M < 0.90
Lean body mass			Increase
Fat mass			Decrease or maintain
Percentage of body fat			Decrease or maintain
pH			Saliva 7.2–7.4
Blood pressure			110/70 to 120/80
Resting heart rate			Decrease

Week 1: Detox

Day 1   Date _____   pH _____

            Weight: _____

Bed Time_____ # hours slept _____ Quality_____	
Breakfast Time _____	**Intake Checklist:** Protein 1 2 3 4
Detox Shake Time _____	Fats 1 2 3 4 Nuts 1
Lunch Time _____	Veggies 1 2 3 4 5 6 7 8 9 10 Fruits 1 2
Detox Shake Time _____	Shakes 1 2
Dinner Time _____	**Hot Hormone Foods:** Olive oil
Water 1 2 3 4 5 6 7 8 9 10 11 12 13 14	Berries Apple
Exercise: Cardio Yoga	Flaxseeds/Chia seeds Broccoli Green Tea **Spices:**
Supplements:	Cinnamon Turmeric Cumin Rosemary
Relaxation:	Oregano Garlic _____ _____

Week 1: Detox

Day 2   Date _____ pH _____

Bed Time_____	# hours slept _____
Quality_____	

Breakfast	**Intake Checklist:**
Time _____	Protein 1 2 3 4
Detox Shake	Fats 1 2 3 4
Time _____	Nuts 1
Lunch	Veggies 1 2 3 4 5 6 7 8 9 10
Time _____	Fruits 1 2
Detox Shake	Shakes 1 2
Time _____	
Dinner	**Hot Hormone Foods:**
Time _____	Olive oil
Water	Berries
1 2 3 4 5 6 7 8 9 10 11 12 13 14	Apple
Exercise:	Flaxseeds/Chia seeds
Cardio	Broccoli
Yoga	Green Tea
	Spices:
Supplements:	Cinnamon
	Turmeric
	Cumin
	Rosemary
Relaxation:	Oregano
	Garlic
	_____
	_____

Week 1: Detox

Day 3   Date _____   pH _____

Bed Time_____   # hours slept _____
Quality_____

Breakfast	Intake Checklist:
Time _____	Protein 1 2 3 4
Detox Shake	Fats 1 2 3 4
Time _____	Nuts 1
Lunch	Veggies 1 2 3 4 5 6 7 8 9 10
Time _____	Fruits 1 2
Detox Shake	Shakes 1 2
Time _____	

Dinner	Hot Hormone Foods:
Time _____	Olive oil
Water	Berries
1 2 3 4 5 6 7 8 9 10 11 12 13 14	Apple
Exercise:	Flaxseeds/Chia seeds
Cardio	Broccoli
Yoga	Green Tea
	Spices:
Supplements:	Cinnamon
	Turmeric
	Cumin
	Rosemary
Relaxation:	Oregano
	Garlic
	_____
	_____

Week 1: Detox

Day 4   Date _____   pH _____

Bed Time_____ # hours slept _____ Quality_____	

Breakfast Time _____	**Intake Checklist:** Protein 1 2 3 4
Detox Shake Time _____	Fats 1 2 3 4 Nuts 1
Lunch Time _____	Veggies 1 2 3 4 5 6 7 8 9 10 Fruits 1 2
Detox Shake Time _____	Shakes 1 2
Dinner Time _____	**Hot Hormone Foods:** Olive oil
Water 1 2 3 4 5 6 7 8 9 10 11 12 13 14	Berries Apple
Exercise: Cardio Yoga	Flaxseeds/Chia seeds Broccoli Green Tea **Spices:**
Supplements:	Cinnamon Turmeric Cumin Rosemary
Relaxation:	Oregano Garlic _____ _____

Week 1: Detox

Day 5   Date _____   pH _____

Bed Time_____ # hours slept _____ Quality_____	
Breakfast Time _____	**Intake Checklist:** Protein 1 2 3 4
Detox Shake Time _____	Fats 1 2 3 4 Nuts 1
Lunch Time _____	Veggies 1 2 3 4 5 6 7 8 9 10 Fruits 1 2
Detox Shake Time _____	Shakes 1 2
Dinner Time _____	**Hot Hormone Foods:** Olive oil
Water 1 2 3 4 5 6 7 8 9 10 11 12 13 14	Berries Apple
Exercise: Cardio Yoga	Flaxseeds/Chia seeds Broccoli Green Tea **Spices:**
Supplements:	Cinnamon Turmeric Cumin Rosemary
Relaxation:	Oregano Garlic _____ _____

Week 1: Detox

Day 6   Date _____   pH _____

Bed Time_____ # hours slept _____ Quality_____	
Breakfast Time _____	**Intake Checklist:** Protein 1 2 3 4
Detox Shake Time _____	Fats 1 2 3 4 Nuts 1
Lunch Time _____	Veggies 1 2 3 4 5 6 7 8 9 10 Fruits 1 2
Detox Shake Time _____	Shakes 1 2
Dinner Time _____	**Hot Hormone Foods:** Olive oil
Water 1 2 3 4 5 6 7 8 9 10 11 12 13 14	Berries Apple
Exercise: Cardio Yoga	Flaxseeds/Chia seeds Broccoli Green Tea **Spices:**
Supplements:	Cinnamon Turmeric Cumin Rosemary
Relaxation:	Oregano Garlic _____ _____

Week 1: Detox

Day 7   Date _____   pH _____

Bed Time_____ # hours slept _____ Quality_____	
Breakfast Time _____	**Intake Checklist:** Protein 1 2 3 4
Detox Shake Time _____	Fats 1 2 3 4 Nuts 1
Lunch Time _____	Veggies 1 2 3 4 5 6 7 8 9 10 Fruits 1 2
Detox Shake Time _____	Shakes 1 2
Dinner Time _____	**Hot Hormone Foods:** Olive oil
Water 1 2 3 4 5 6 7 8 9 10 11 12 13 14	Berries Apple
Exercise: Cardio Yoga	Flaxseeds/Chia seeds Broccoli Green Tea **Spices:**
Supplements:	Cinnamon Turmeric Cumin Rosemary
Relaxation:	Oregano Garlic _____ _____

Week 2: Detox

Day 1   Date _____   pH _____
               Weight: _____

Bed Time_____ # hours slept _____ Quality_____	

Breakfast Time _____	**Intake Checklist:** Protein 1 2 3 4
Detox Shake Time _____	Fats 1 2 3 4 Nuts 1 2
Lunch Time _____	Veggies 1 2 3 4 5 6 7 8 9 10 Fruits 1 2
Detox Shake Time _____	Shakes 1 2 Gluten-free Grain/Potato 1
Dinner Time _____	**Hot Hormone Foods:** Olive oil
Water 1 2 3 4 5 6 7 8 9 10 11 12 13 14	Berries Apple
Exercise: Cardio Yoga	Flaxseeds/Chia seeds Broccoli Green Tea **Spices:**
Supplements:	Cinnamon Turmeric Cumin Rosemary
Relaxation:	Oregano Garlic _____ _____

Week 2: Detox

Day 2   Date _____   pH _____

Bed Time_____ # hours slept _____ Quality_____	
Breakfast Time _____	**Intake Checklist:** Protein 1 2 3 4
Detox Shake Time _____	Fats 1 2 3 4 Nuts 1 2
Lunch Time _____	Veggies 1 2 3 4 5 6 7 8 9 10 Fruits 1 2
Detox Shake Time _____	Shakes 1 2 Gluten-free Grain/Potato 1
Dinner Time _____	**Hot Hormone Foods:** Olive oil
Water 1 2 3 4 5 6 7 8 9 10 11 12 13 14	Berries Apple
Exercise: Cardio Yoga	Flaxseeds/Chia seeds Broccoli Green Tea **Spices:**
Supplements:	Cinnamon Turmeric Cumin Rosemary
Relaxation:	Oregano Garlic _____ _____

Week 2: Detox

Day 3   Date _____ pH _____

Bed Time_____ # hours slept _____ Quality_____	
Breakfast Time _____	**Intake Checklist:** Protein 1 2 3 4
Detox Shake Time _____	Fats 1 2 3 4 Nuts 1 2
Lunch Time _____	Veggies 1 2 3 4 5 6 7 8 9 10 Fruits 1 2
Detox Shake Time _____	Shakes 1 2 Gluten-free Grain/Potato 1
Dinner Time _____	**Hot Hormone Foods:** Olive oil
Water 1 2 3 4 5 6 7 8 9 10 11 12 13 14	Berries Apple
Exercise: Cardio Yoga	Flaxseeds/Chia seeds Broccoli Green Tea **Spices:**
Supplements:	Cinnamon Turmeric Cumin Rosemary
Relaxation:	Oregano Garlic _____ _____

Week 2: Detox

Day 4   Date _____   pH _____

Bed Time_____ # hours slept _____ Quality_____	
Breakfast Time _____	**Intake Checklist:** Protein 1 2 3 4
Detox Shake Time _____	Fats 1 2 3 4 Nuts 1 2
Lunch Time _____	Veggies 1 2 3 4 5 6 7 8 9 10 Fruits 1 2
Detox Shake Time _____	Shakes 1 2 Gluten-free Grain/Potato 1
Dinner Time _____	**Hot Hormone Foods:** Olive oil
Water 1 2 3 4 5 6 7 8 9 10 11 12 13 14	Berries Apple
Exercise: Cardio Yoga	Flaxseeds/Chia seeds Broccoli Green Tea **Spices:**
Supplements:	Cinnamon Turmeric Cumin Rosemary
Relaxation:	Oregano Garlic _____ _____

Week 2: Detox

Day 5   Date _____   pH _____

Bed Time_____ # hours slept _____ Quality_____	
Breakfast Time _____	**Intake Checklist:** Protein 1 2 3 4
Detox Shake Time _____	Fats 1 2 3 4 Nuts 1 2
Lunch Time _____	Veggies 1 2 3 4 5 6 7 8 9 10 Fruits 1 2
Detox Shake Time _____	Shakes 1 2 Gluten-free Grain/Potato 1
Dinner Time _____	**Hot Hormone Foods:** Olive oil
Water 1 2 3 4 5 6 7 8 9 10 11 12 13 14	Berries Apple
Exercise: Cardio Yoga	Flaxseeds/Chia seeds Broccoli Green Tea **Spices:**
Supplements:	Cinnamon Turmeric Cumin Rosemary
Relaxation:	Oregano Garlic _____ _____

Week 2: Detox

Day 6   Date _____   pH _____

Bed Time_____   # hours slept _____
Quality_____

Breakfast Time _____	**Intake Checklist:** Protein 1 2 3 4
Detox Shake Time _____	Fats 1 2 3 4 Nuts 1 2
Lunch Time _____	Veggies 1 2 3 4 5 6 7 8 9 10 Fruits 1 2
Detox Shake Time _____	Shakes 1 2 Gluten-free Grain/Potato 1
Dinner Time _____	**Hot Hormone Foods:** Olive oil
Water 1 2 3 4 5 6 7 8 9 10 11 12 13 14	Berries Apple
Exercise: Cardio Yoga	Flaxseeds/Chia seeds Broccoli Green Tea **Spices:**
Supplements:	Cinnamon Turmeric Cumin Rosemary
Relaxation:	Oregano Garlic _____ _____

Week 2: Detox

Day 7   Date _____   pH _____

Bed Time_____ # hours slept _____ Quality_____	
Breakfast Time _____	**Intake Checklist:** Protein 1 2 3 4
Detox Shake Time _____	Fats 1 2 3 4 Nuts 1 2
Lunch Time _____	Veggies 1 2 3 4 5 6 7 8 9 10 Fruits 1 2
Detox Shake Time _____	Shakes 1 2 Gluten-free Grain/Potato 1
Dinner Time _____	**Hot Hormone Foods:** Olive oil
Water 1 2 3 4 5 6 7 8 9 10 11 12 13 14	Berries Apple
Exercise: Cardio Yoga	Flaxseeds/Chia seeds Broccoli Green Tea **Spices:**
Supplements:	Cinnamon Turmeric Cumin Rosemary
Relaxation:	Oregano Garlic _____ _____

Week 3: Transition Week

Day 1   Date _____   pH _____
               Weight: _____

Bed Time_____ # hours slept _____ Quality_____	
Breakfast Time _____	**Intake Checklist:** Protein 1 2 3 4
Detox Shake Time _____	Fats 1 2 3 4 Nuts 1 2
Lunch Time _____	Veggies 1 2 3 4 5 6 7 8 9 10 Fruits 1 2
Detox Shake Time _____	Shakes 1 2 Test Food 1
Dinner Time _____	**Test Food for Today:**
Water 1 2 3 4 5 6 7 8 9 10 11 12 13 14	**Symptoms Noted:**
Exercise: Cardio Yoga	
Supplements:	
Relaxation:	

Week 3: Transition Week

Day 2   Date _____   pH _____

Bed Time_____   # hours slept _____

Quality_____

Breakfast Time _____	**Intake Checklist:** Protein 1 2 3 4
Detox Shake Time _____	Fats 1 2 3 4 Nuts 1 2
Lunch Time _____	Veggies 1 2 3 4 5 6 7 8 9 10 Fruits 1 2
Detox Shake Time _____	Shakes 1 2 Test Food 1
Dinner Time _____	**Test Food for Today:**
Water 1 2 3 4 5 6 7 8 9 10 11 12 13 14	**Symptoms Noted:**
Exercise: Cardio Yoga	
Supplements:	
Relaxation:	

Week 3: Transition Week

Day 3   Date _____   pH _____

Bed Time_____ # hours slept _____ Quality_____	
Breakfast Time _____	**Intake Checklist:** Protein 1 2 3 4
Detox Shake Time _____	Fats 1 2 3 4 Nuts 1 2
Lunch Time _____	Veggies 1 2 3 4 5 6 7 8 9 10 Fruits 1 2
Detox Shake Time _____	Shakes 1 2 Test Food 1
Dinner Time _____	**Test Food for Today:**
Water 1 2 3 4 5 6 7 8 9 10 11 12 13 14	**Symptoms Noted:**
Exercise: Cardio Yoga	
Supplements:	
Relaxation:	

Week 3: Transition Week

Day 4   Date _____   pH _____

Bed Time_____ # hours slept _____ Quality_____	
Breakfast Time _____	**Intake Checklist:** Protein 1 2 3 4
Detox Shake Time _____	Fats 1 2 3 4 Nuts 1 2
Lunch Time _____	Veggies 1 2 3 4 5 6 7 8 9 10 Fruits 1 2
Detox Shake Time _____	Shakes 1 2 Test Food 1
Dinner Time _____	**Test Food for Today:**
Water 1 2 3 4 5 6 7 8 9 10 11 12 13 14	**Symptoms Noted:**
Exercise: Cardio Yoga	
Supplements:	
Relaxation:	

Week 3: Transition Week

Day 5   Date _____   pH _____

Bed Time_____ # hours slept _____ Quality_____	
Breakfast Time _____	**Intake Checklist:** Protein 1 2 3 4
Detox Shake Time _____	Fats 1 2 3 4 Nuts 1 2
Lunch Time _____	Veggies 1 2 3 4 5 6 7 8 9 10 Fruits 1 2
Detox Shake Time _____	Shakes 1 2 Test Food 1
Dinner Time _____	**Test Food for Today:**
Water 1 2 3 4 5 6 7 8 9 10 11 12 13 14	**Symptoms Noted:**
Exercise: Cardio Yoga	
Supplements:	
Relaxation:	

Week 3: Transition Week

Day 6   Date _____   pH _____

Bed Time_____ # hours slept _____ Quality_____	
Breakfast Time _____	**Intake Checklist:** Protein 1 2 3 4
Detox Shake Time _____	Fats 1 2 3 4 Nuts 1 2
Lunch Time _____	Veggies 1 2 3 4 5 6 7 8 9 10 Fruits 1 2
Detox Shake Time _____	Shakes 1 2 Test Food 1
Dinner Time _____	**Test Food for Today:**
Water 1 2 3 4 5 6 7 8 9 10 11 12 13 14	**Symptoms Noted:**
Exercise: Cardio Yoga	
Supplements:	
Relaxation:	

Week 3: Transition Week

Day 7   Date _____ pH _____

Bed Time_____   # hours slept _____
Quality_____

Breakfast	Intake Checklist:
Time _____	Protein 1 2 3 4
Detox Shake	Fats 1 2 3 4
Time _____	Nuts 1 2
Lunch	Veggies 1 2 3 4 5 6 7 8 9 10
Time _____	Fruits 1 2
Detox Shake	Shakes 1 2
Time _____	Test Food 1
Dinner	**Test Food for Today:**
Time _____	
Water	
1 2 3 4 5 6 7 8 9 10 11 12 13 14	**Symptoms Noted:**
Exercise:	
Cardio	
Yoga	
Supplements:	
Relaxation:	

Week 4: The Glyci-Med Approach

Day 1   Date _____ pH _____
             Weight: _____

Bed Time_____ # hours slept _____ Quality_____	
Breakfast Time _____	**Intake Checklist:** Protein 1 2 3 4
Detox Shake Time _____	Fats 1 2 3 4 Nuts 1 2
Lunch Time _____	Veggies 1 2 3 4 5 6 7 8 9 10 Fruits 1 2
Detox Shake Time _____	Shakes 1 2 Starchy Veg/Grain/Potato 1 Dairy 1
Dinner Time _____	**Hot Hormone Foods:** Olive oil
Water 1 2 3 4 5 6 7 8 9 10 11 12 13 14	Berries Apple
Exercise: Cardio Yoga	Flaxseeds/Chia seeds Broccoli Green Tea **Spices:**
Supplements:	Cinnamon Turmeric Cumin Rosemary
Relaxation:	Oregano Garlic _____ _____

Week 4: The Glyci-Med Approach

Day 2   Date _____   pH _____

Bed Time_____ # hours slept _____ Quality_____	

Breakfast Time _____	**Intake Checklist:** Protein 1 2 3 4
Detox Shake Time _____	Fats 1 2 3 4 Nuts 1 2
Lunch Time _____	Veggies 1 2 3 4 5 6 7 8 9 10 Fruits 1 2
Detox Shake Time _____	Shakes 1 2 Starchy Veg/Grain/Potato 1 Dairy 1
Dinner Time _____	**Hot Hormone Foods:** Olive oil
Water 1 2 3 4 5 6 7 8 9 10 11 12 13 14	Berries Apple
Exercise: Cardio Yoga	Flaxseeds/Chia seeds Broccoli Green Tea **Spices:**
Supplements:	Cinnamon Turmeric Cumin Rosemary
Relaxation:	Oregano Garlic _____ _____

Week 4: The Glyci-Med Approach

Day 3   Date _____   pH _____

Bed Time_____   # hours slept _____
Quality_____

Breakfast	Intake Checklist:
Time _____	Protein 1 2 3 4
Detox Shake	Fats 1 2 3 4
Time _____	Nuts 1 2
Lunch	Veggies 1 2 3 4 5 6 7 8 9 10
Time _____	Fruits 1 2
	Shakes 1 2
Detox Shake	Starchy Veg/Grain/Potato 1
Time _____	Dairy 1

Dinner	Hot Hormone Foods:
Time _____	Olive oil
Water	Berries
1 2 3 4 5 6 7 8 9 10 11 12 13 14	Apple
Exercise:	Flaxseeds/Chia seeds
Cardio	Broccoli
Yoga	Green Tea
	Spices:
Supplements:	Cinnamon
	Turmeric
	Cumin
	Rosemary
Relaxation:	Oregano
	Garlic
	_____
	_____

Week 4: The Glyci-Med Approach

Day 4   Date _____   pH _____

Bed Time_____ # hours slept _____	
Quality_____	

Breakfast	Intake Checklist:
Time _____	Protein 1 2 3 4
Detox Shake	Fats 1 2 3 4
Time _____	Nuts 1 2
Lunch	Veggies 1 2 3 4 5 6 7 8 9 10
Time _____	Fruits 1 2
	Shakes 1 2
Detox Shake	Starchy Veg/Grain/Potato 1
Time _____	Dairy 1
Dinner	**Hot Hormone Foods:**
Time _____	Olive oil
Water	Berries
1 2 3 4 5 6 7 8 9 10 11 12 13 14	Apple
Exercise:	Flaxseeds/Chia seeds
Cardio	Broccoli
Yoga	Green Tea
	Spices:
Supplements:	Cinnamon
	Turmeric
	Cumin
	Rosemary
Relaxation:	Oregano
	Garlic
	_____
	_____

Week 4: The Glyci-Med Approach

Day 5   Date _____   pH _____

Bed Time_____	# hours slept _____
Quality_____	

Breakfast	**Intake Checklist:**
Time _____	Protein 1 2 3 4
Detox Shake	Fats 1 2 3 4
Time _____	Nuts 1 2
Lunch	Veggies 1 2 3 4 5 6 7 8 9 10
Time _____	Fruits 1 2
	Shakes 1 2
Detox Shake	Starchy Veg/Grain/Potato 1
Time _____	Dairy 1
Dinner	**Hot Hormone Foods:**
Time _____	Olive oil
Water	Berries
1 2 3 4 5 6 7 8 9 10 11 12 13 14	Apple
Exercise:	Flaxseeds/Chia seeds
Cardio	Broccoli
Yoga	Green Tea
	Spices:
Supplements:	Cinnamon
	Turmeric
	Cumin
	Rosemary
	Oregano
Relaxation:	Garlic
	_____
	_____

Week 4: The Glyci-Med Approach

Day 6   Date _____   pH _____

Bed Time _____ # hours slept _____ Quality _____	
Breakfast Time _____	**Intake Checklist:** Protein 1 2 3 4
Detox Shake Time _____	Fats 1 2 3 4 Nuts 1 2
Lunch Time _____	Veggies 1 2 3 4 5 6 7 8 9 10 Fruits 1 2
Detox Shake Time _____	Shakes 1 2 Starchy Veg/Grain/Potato 1 Dairy 1
Dinner Time _____	**Hot Hormone Foods:** Olive oil
Water 1 2 3 4 5 6 7 8 9 10 11 12 13 14	Berries Apple
Exercise: Cardio Yoga	Flaxseeds/Chia seeds Broccoli Green Tea **Spices:**
Supplements:	Cinnamon Turmeric Cumin Rosemary
Relaxation:	Oregano Garlic _____ _____

Week 4: The Glyci-Med Approach

Day 7   Date _____   pH _____

Bed Time_____   # hours slept _____
Quality_____

Breakfast	**Intake Checklist:**
Time _____	Protein 1 2 3 4
Detox Shake	Fats 1 2 3 4
Time _____	Nuts 1 2
Lunch	Veggies 1 2 3 4 5 6 7 8 9 10
Time _____	Fruits 1 2
	Shakes 1 2
Detox Shake	Starchy Veg/Grain/Potato 1
Time _____	Dairy 1
Dinner	**Hot Hormone Foods:**
Time _____	Olive oil
Water	Berries
1 2 3 4 5 6 7 8 9 10 11 12 13 14	Apple
Exercise:	Flaxseeds/Chia seeds
Cardio	Broccoli
Yoga	Green Tea
	Spices:
Supplements:	Cinnamon
	Turmeric
	Cumin
	Rosemary
Relaxation:	Oregano
	Garlic
	_____
	_____

ACKNOWLEDGMENTS

Thank you to my family and friends for supporting my work. I could never achieve all that I do without your help.

My sincerest gratitude to Andrea Ritter for her editing skills, and to Tara Rose for your help with *every* project that I take on—you are an amazing asset, a caring person, and a fabulous right-hand woman! And to the team of practitioners and staff at Clear Medicine—I am so blessed to work with all of you. To Natalie Shay, thank you so much for taking the time to read this manuscript and offer your feedback, and for your unbelievable ongoing support.

Thank you to my agent Rick Broadhead for your input, sales efforts and highly principled work ethic. I am lucky to have you. Thank you to Rodale—specifically Aly Mostel and Lauren Harvey—for promoting *The Hormone Diet* and *The Carb Sensitivity Program*. I would also like to thank Dr. Mehmet Oz, Suzanne Somers (*Sexy Forever*) and Dr. William Davis (*Wheat Belly* and *Lose the Wheat, Lose the Weight*) for their continued support of my work.

Lastly, thank you to my patients and to the readers and followers of the original *Hormone Diet*. Without you taking the time to offer your suggestions, this book would not have come into existence.

RESOURCES

Heavy Metal Detox:
Detoxamin: EDTA suppositories: detoxamin.com

Infrared Sauna:
SaunaRay Far Infrared Saunas: saunaray.com

Natural Lubricants:
Hathor: hathorbody.com
O'My: omyinternational.com

Body Fat/Composition Analyzer:
Tanita: Home body-fat analyzer: tanita.com

Light Therapy
Yumalite: Head-mounted light visor: yumalite.com (Discount code: NTYUMA)

Natural Skin Care and Makeup:
Naturopathica: Environmental Defense Facial Mask:
      naturopathica.com
Be.Products Company: Skin care made from natural food: befine.com
Caudalie: (Toxin free skin care): http://us.caudalie.com
Juice Beauty: (Toxin free skin care): juicebeauty.com
John Masters: (Toxin free skin and hair care): johnmasters.com;
      drnatashaturner.com or clearmedicine.com
Burt's Bees: Natural skin care: burtsbees.com
Alba Organics: Sugar Cane Body Polish, Kukui Nut Organic Body Oil:
      albaorganics.com (Unlike the two products listed here, all Alba
      products are *not* free of harmful methylparabens and propylparabens.)
Sephora: (Options for organic, toxin free skin care): sephora.com
Dr. Hauschka Skin Care: drhauschka.com
Jane Iredale: Mineral makeup: janeiredale.com

Supplements:
Xymogen: xymogen.com or clearmedicine.com
Douglas Laboratories: douglaslabs.com or clearmedicine.com

Wobenzym N: One of the top-selling natural anti-inflammatory enzyme formulas in the world: wobenzym-usa.com; drnatashaturner.com or clearmedicine.com

All Clear Medicine Products, including those for detoxification, general health and hormonal concerns: clearmedicine.com or drnatashaturner.com

Carlson Fish Oils: carlsonlabs.com

Nordic Natural Fish Oils : nordicnaturals.com

Jarrow: jarrow.com

Genuine Health: (Proteins +, all natural whey protein isolate supplement and Greens +, green food supplements): genuinehealth.com

New Chapter: newchapter.com

AOR: aorhealth.com; drnatashaturner.com or clearmedicine.com

Dream Protein (all natural whey protein supplement): drnatashaturner.com or clearmedicine.com

Pure Encapsulations: (G.I. Fortify and Liver G.I. Detox): pureencapsulations.com; drnatashaturner.com or clearmedicine.com

Metagenics: metagenics.com; drnatashaturner.com or clearmedicine.com

Specialty Foods:

Maranatha: all natural nut butters: maranathafoods.com

Artisana: Organic food options, including coconut butter and raw nut butters: artisanafoods.com

Navitas Naturals: organic superfoods from acai powder to cocao powder: navitasnaturals.com

Muir Glen Organic: premium, quality organic sauces and salsas: muirglen.com

Frontera Salsa: gourmet, organic salsa: fronterafiesta.com

Redwood Hills: great tasting goat milk products: redwoodhill.com

Edensoy: organic soy milk, beans, soups, teas and more: edenfoods.com

Cabot Cheese: High protein, lactose-free cheese options: cabotcheese.coop

Chobani: Greek yogurt with natural ingredients: chobani.com

Organic Valley: organic dairy products: organicvalley.coop

Horizon Organic: organic dairy products: horizondairy.com

Cruncha ma-me: Edemame snacks: crunchamame.com

Crystal Farms: 100 percent egg whites: allwhiteseggwhites.com

Fage: Tasty Greek yogurt options: usa.fage.eu

Green and Black's: Organic chocolate: greenandblacks.com

NewTree: Fine Belgian dark chocolate: newtree.com

The Simply Bar: Gluten-free protein bar: thesimplybar.com; drnatashaturner.com or clearmedicine.com

Sambazon: Açaí concentrate: sambazon.com
Navitas Naturals: Goji Powder: navitasnaturals.com
POM Wonderful: Pomegranate juice: pomwonderful.com
La Tortilla Factory: Pita, wraps and gluten-free products: latortillafactory.com
Aiya Teas: Green tea: aiya-america.com
Xylitol: Low-glycemic treats: xylitolusa.com
Quest: Low-carb, gluten-free protein bars: questproteinbar.com
Food for Life Baking Co.: Ezekiel breads: foodforlife.com
Bob's Red Mill Natural Foods: Gluten-free and other grain products: bobsredmill.com
PROsnack Natural Foods: Elevate Me! (organic whole-food and protein bar): prosnack.com

Mineralized Alkaline Water Products:
Santevia: santevia.com

Toxin-Free Household Cleaning Products:
NatureClean: naturecleanliving.com
Attitude: cleanattitude.com
Seventh Generation: seventhgeneration.com

Organic Cotton Bedding and Mattresses:
The Guide to Less Toxic Products: lesstoxicguide.ca

Health Information Resources:
Pharmacy Compounding Accreditation Board (PCAB): Find a compounding pharmacy in your area. pcab.org/accredited-pharmacies
Alive Magazine: Natural health magazine. alive.com
Life Extension Foundation: lef.org
Mary Shomon's thyroid health website: thyroid.about.com
SeaChoice: Healthy seafood choices: seachoice.org
Harvard School of Public Health: The Nutrition Source hsph.harvard.edu/nutritionsource/index.html
Whole Foods Market: Tasty soup recipes!: wholefoodsmarket.com/recipes
Trader Joe's: recipes and more: traderjoes.com/recipes
Environmental Working Group: Information about cosmetics, seafood safety, etc.: ewg.org
Calorie King: Nutrition information database: calorieking.com
Glycemic Index and GI Database (AU): glycemicindex.com
American Journal of Clinical Nutrition Glycemic Load Chart: ajcn.org/cgi/content/full/76/1/5#SEC2
International Hormone Society: intlhormonesociety.org

GENERAL INDEX

Underscored page references indicate boxed text. **Boldface** references indicate illustrations.

Abdominal fat, 18—20, 43, 85, 157
Açaí berries, 106–7
Acetylcholine, 14, 184–85, 213–14
Acetyl-L-carnitine, 213
Acidic body pH, 45–46, 330
Acid reflux, 27, 72, 74
Acrylamide, 71
Addiction, to food, 23
Adiponectin, 101, 191
Adrenal gland fatigue, 201–2
Adrenaline, 12, 19, 20, 84
Aerobic workouts, 160
Aging, 164, 167
Agricultural hormone use, 33–35
Air conditioning, effects of, 167–68
Alcohol
    carbohydrates and, 95
    in detox phase, 60
    effects of, 25, 90, 167
    sensitivity testing, 254
Alkaline body pH, 45–46, 330
Allergies. See Food intolerance/sensitivity
Almond butter, 121–22
Almond milk, 62, 131, 133, 231, 232
Almonds, 104
Aloe vera, 69, 73
Alpha-lipoic acid, 192
Amino acid supplements, 215
Anabolic steroids, in food production, 33
Anandamide, 111
Andropause, 208
Angelica, 206
Anise, 73
Antacids, 72–73
Anthocyanins, 106
Antibiotics, 34, 76–77
Antidepressant medications, 35, 156, 195
Antifungal agents, 77
Anti-inflammatory foods, 143–44
Antioxidants, 52

Anxiety, 7, 165
Appetite
    control of, 89
    digestive health role, 67
    factors in, 14–15, 164, 166–67, 167–68
Apple cider vinegar, 123
Apples, 69, 89, 102–3, 155
Arginine, 209, 215
Artichoke, 69, 218
Artificial sweeteners, 25, 60–61, 64, 91, 94
Ashwagandha, 162, 199–200, 211
Aspartame, 91
Assessment. See Tracking
Avocados, 101–2, 278
Awareness, meditation and, 84

Bacteria. See Gut flora
Basal metabolic rate, 166
Beans
    in detox plan, 62, 240–41, 250–51
    serving sizes, 270, 272, 274
Bedtime, timing of, 57–58
Beef, 33–34, 191
Beet leaf, 69
Beets, 69
Benchmarking tests
    list of, 226–28
    overview, 217–18
    test descriptions, 218–26
Berberine, 74, 77
Berries, 94, 106–7, 155
Best Body Assessment, 39–49
Beta-sitosterol, 102, 104
Beverages. See also specific beverages
    serving sizes, 278
    shopping tips, 130–33, 132
    timing of intake, 55
    tracking of, 329
Bezwecken, 201

hormonal health profile
checklists, 174–86
Treatment Pyramid, 186–88, **187**
produced in digestive tract, 26–29, 53
sleep and, 54–58
testing of, 222–28
Hot Hormone foods, 98–111
HRT (hormone replacement therapy), 35
Hydrochloric acid supplements, 74
Hydrocortisone, 201
Hydrolyzed milk protein, 200, 208
Hypoglycemia, 51
Hypothyroidism, 9–10, 225–26

IBS (Irritable Bowel Syndrome), 27
IGF-I (insulin-like growth factor I), 34, 226
Immune system, 62, 202
Indole-3-carbinol (I3C), 98, 204
Inflammation
diet and, 24, 109–10
effects of, 6
in hormonal health profile, 174–75
obesity role, 12
supplement recommendations, 188–90
yoga's effects on, 84–85
Ingredient labels, 114
Inositol, 52, 144, 196
Insulin levels
balancing (*see* Insulin sensitivity)
diet and, 87–88, 106
excess (*see* Insulin resistance)
testing of, 219–20
testosterone levels and, 210
Insulin-like growth factor I (IGF-I), 34, 226
Insulin resistance
effects of, 6, 7, 10, 19–20
in hormonal health profile, 175–76
supplement recommendations,
190–93
Insulin sensitivity
adiponectin effects, 191
diet and, 22–23, 101, 107
muscle and, 42
sleep deprivation effects, 165
Interleukin-6, 85
Interval training, 159–60
Intolerance. *See* Food intolerance/
sensitivity
Iodine, 212
Iron, 103, 107
Irritable Bowel Syndrome (IBS), 27

Isocort, 201
Isothiocyanates, 98
I3C (indole-3-carbinol), 98, 204

Jet lag, 167
Joint pain, 254
Juice, 95, 130–31, 278

Kamut, 253, 254, 259
Kitchen equipment, toxins in, 65. *See also*
Cooking tips

Label-reading tips, 114–16
Lactobacillus acidophilus, 75–77
Lactose intolerance, 27
L-alpha-glycerophosphocholine, 213–14
LDL, testing of, 220–21
Lean body mass, 41
Leptin, 57, 96, 101, 104
L-glutamine, 144
LH (Lutenizing Hormone), 223
Licorice, 69, 73, 201, 206
Lifestyle changes, 46
Light exposure, 55, 56–57, 165
Lignans, 99
Lipoic acid, 52
Liver function
detoxification role, 31, 35, 51–52, 211
herbal cleansing formulas, 69
testing of, 218
Low-fat diets, 87
L-tyrosine, 156, 193, 212
Lunch recipes, 291–99
Lutenizing Hormone (LH), 223
Lysine, 215

Macronutrient ratio
failure to balance, 26
label-reading tips, 115
meal planning for, 92–95
nuts and, 104
overview, 88–89, 117, 168–69
Magnesium
benefits, 46, 52
sources of, 103, 107, 108
supplements, 66, 73, 162, 192,
197–98, 204
Mahi mahi, 135–36
Male menopause, 208
Manganese, 107
Margarine, 64

Marshmallow, 69, 73
Mastica gum, 74
Mayonnaise, 122, <u>278</u>
Meal planning. *See also Supercharged
    Hormone Diet*
    macronutrient ratio in, 92–95
    timing of meals/snacks, <u>26</u>, <u>54–55</u>,
        90–91
Measurement. *See* Tracking
Meat
    in detox plan, 61, 62, <u>240–41</u>, <u>250–51</u>
    hormone imbalance role, <u>24</u>
    organic sources, 92
    sensitivity testing, <u>254</u>
    shopping tips, 133–34
Medications, as toxins, 35–36
Meditation, benefits of, <u>82–84</u>
Mediterranean diet, 87, 88
Melatonin
    appetite and, <u>14</u>
    foods/habits affecting, 59, 166, 214
    hormonal health profile, <u>185</u>
    precursors, 103
    sleep and, 21, <u>57</u>
    sources of, 104
    supplements, 163, 214
Memory, serotonin and, 7
Menopause, 8–9, <u>151</u>, 205–7
Metabolic Repair Pack, 190, 192, 221
Metabolic Syndrome, 20
Metabolism
    basal rate, 166
    body temperature and, <u>167–68</u>
    boosting, 154
    diet and, 31–32, 58–59, 90, 99
    environmental toxins and, 30
    hormone stimulation of, <u>12–13</u>
    muscle and, <u>42</u>, 156–60
    resting rate, 160
Methionine, 52
Milk alternatives, 62, 131, 133, <u>276</u>
Milk production, hormone use in, 34
Milk protein hydrolysate, 200, 208
Milk thistle, 69, 204, 218
Mindfulness, <u>84</u>
Mineral supplements, 192–93
Monounsaturated fats, 87, 100–101, 102
Mood
    food sensitivity symptoms, <u>61</u>, <u>254</u>
    serotonin and, 7
    sleep deprivation effects, <u>164</u>

Motivation, 46–49
Muscle
    growth/development of, <u>13–14</u>, <u>42</u>,
        156–60
    metabolically active, 19
    wasting of, 198
Mushrooms, 76

Nasal symptoms, of food intolerance/
        sensitivity, <u>62</u>, 254
Nattokinase, 189
Nervous system, 28, 144
Neurology. *See* Cognitive function
Noradrenaline, <u>12</u>, <u>56</u>
Nut butters, 121–22, 155
Nutrition labels, 114–16
Nuts
    benefits, 104
    in detox plan, 62, <u>240–41</u>, <u>250–51</u>
    in Glyci-Med approach, 89
    serving sizes, <u>272</u>
    as snack, 155
Nystatin, 77

Oat milk, 62
Oats/oat bran, 107, 119–20
Obesity and overweight, 6, 20–21, 24
Oils
    in detox plan, 60, 62, <u>240–41</u>, <u>250–51</u>
    extra-virgin olive oil, 60, 89, 100–101,
        <u>278</u>
    serving sizes, <u>278</u>
    unhealthy types, 101, 117, <u>279</u>
Olive leaf extract, 77
Olive oil, extra-virgin, 60, 89, 100–101, <u>278</u>
Olives, <u>278</u>
Omega-3 fatty acids, 103
Oranges, 253, <u>254</u>
Oregano oil, 74, 77
Organic foods, 34, 89, 92, 103, 105
Ornithine, 215
Overeating, <u>25</u>
Overexercising, 46, 80–81, 157
Oxygen consumption, 160

Packaged foods, <u>64</u>, 91. *See also*
        Shopping tips
Pain sensitivity, <u>83–84</u>, <u>164–65</u>
Partially hydrogenated oils, 60, <u>64</u>, 117
Passionflower, 197
Pasta, 93, 121, 262

PCOS (polycystic ovary syndrome), 210, 223
Peanuts, 60, 91
Pecans, 104
Peptic ulcers, 27, 72
Peptide YY, 67
Pesticides, 8, 102
pH balance, 46–47, 330
Phenylalanine, 193–94
Phenylethylamine, 110
Phosphatidylcholine, 82
Phosphatidylserine (PS), 200, 213
Phthalates, 9, 30, 71
Phytoestrogens, 105, 205–6
Pickles, 122
Pizza, 94
Plantains, 73
Plastic containers, 65
Polycystic ovary syndrome (PCOS),
    210, 223
Polyphenols, 99, 100
Pomegranates, 109
Portion control. See Serving sizes
Potassium, 46, 102, 103, 131
Potatoes, 60, 63, 241, 250–51
Poultry, serving sizes, 276
Pregnancy, 213
Premenopause, 203–4, 227–28
Priority, health as, 5
Probiotics, 68, 76–77, 108
Processed foods, 64, 91
Progesterone
    in food supply, 34
    hormonal health profile, 181–82
    metabolism effects, 13
    supplement recommendations, 207–8
    testing of, 225
Prostate cancer, 109
Protein. See also Macronutrient ratio
    appetite and, 67
    benefits, 58–59
    daily intake recommendations, 116
    on nutrition labels, 115
    serving sizes, 276
    in smoothies, 142–43
    sources of, 103, 107, 108
Protein bars, 136
Protein powders, 136–38. See also Whey
    protein isolate
PS (phosphatidylserine), 200, 213
Psyllium, 69
Puncture vine, 209

Quercetin, 102, 109

Raisins, 92
rbGH, 34
Red clover, 206
Red rice yeast extract, 221
Reintroduction, of foods, 253–61
Relationships, sleep deprivation effects, 164
Relaxation habits, 330
Relora, 161–62, 199, 202
Reproductive/fertility issues, 13, 29, 30,
    144, 211
Resistance training, 156–60
Restaurant dining, tips for, 138–39,
    139–40
Resting metabolic rate (RMR), 160
Resveratrim, 191
Resveratrol, 100, 190–91
Reverse-osmosis filtering systems, 65, 105
Rhodiola, 194, 195–96, 200, 212
Rice, 93, 262
RMR (resting metabolic rate), 160
Room temperature, sleep quality and, 56
Rosemary, 109
Rosemary extract, 204
Rutin, 108
Rye, 253, 254, 258

Safflower oil, 60
Sage, 206
St. John's Wort, 196
Saliva hormone analysis, 222–23
Salmon, shopping tips, 91, 135
Salsa, 124
Sandwiches, alternatives to, 93
Sashimi, 93
Saturated fats, 87, 92
Sauces
    recipes, 323–24
    shopping tips, 124–25, 124
Saw palmetto, 210
Seafood. See Fish and seafood
Seasoning mixes, 123
Seeds
    in detox plan, 62, 240, 250–51
    as snack, 155
Selenium, 104, 107, 212–13
Sensitivity. See Food intolerance/sensitivity
Serotonin
    activity of, 144
    appetite and, 14

Serotonin (*cont.*)
   effects of, 7, 110, 194–95
   estrogen and, 225
   foods/habits affecting, 22–23, 59, 93, 106, 196
   hormonal health profile, 176–77
   precursors, 103, 110
   sleep quality and, 57
   supplement recommendations, 195–96
Serving sizes
   in Glyci-Med approach, 89
   on labels, 114–15, 116, 116
   in restaurants, 138–39
   table of, 270–79
7-Keto DHEA, 202–3
Shakes, for detox, 231–32, 262
Sheep's milk cheese, 60
Shift work, 21, 167
Shopping tips
   beverages, 130–33, 132
   breads/pasta/flours, 120–21
   cereals, 118–19
   condiments, 122–24, 125
   dairy products, 127–28
   meats/vegetarian proteins, 133–35
   overview, 113–17
   protein bars/powder, 136–38
   sauces/flavorings, 124–25
   spreads/dips, 125
   sweeteners, 118
   treats, 129–30
Shortening, 64
Skin health, 61, 71, 164, 213
Sleep habits
   disruption of, 20–21, 24, 54–58, 163–65
   improved, tips for, 162–63, 214
   tracking of, 330
Slippery elm, 73
Smoothies
   base ingredients, 142–44
   Detox Shakes, 231–32, 262
   recipes for, 145–51
Snacks
   macronutrient ratio in, 116
   recommendations for, 154–55, 230–32
   shopping tips, 126–27, 129–30
Soda, 23, 131, 132
Sodium, 116
Soluble fiber, 69–70

Soups, 94
Soy products
   benefits, 105
   in detox plan, 62, 240, 250–51
   fermented, 137, 205
   milk, 131–32
   oil, 101, 117
Soy sauce, 122
Spices
   benefits, 109–10
   in detox plan, 240–41, 250–51
   seasoning mixes, 123
   serving sizes, 278
Spreads, shopping tips, 125
Steroid hormones, 33, 34
Stevia, 63
Stomach acid, 72–73
Stomach upset, 27, 72
Strength training, 156–60
Stress
   from calorie restriction, 31
   chronic, effects of, 8, 18–20
   cortisol and, 8, 12, 19–20, 161, 198
   eating habits and, 26
   exercise and, 81, 84–85, 158–59
   management tips, 161–62, 198
Success stories
   adrenal support, 140–41
   healthy habits, 37–38, 79, 86, 112
   hormone balance, 216
   inflammation, 96–97
   mood issues, 151–52
   weight control/loss, 50, 172
Sugar
   as forbidden food, 60–61
   hidden sources of, 132
   neurological effects, 22–23
   sensitivity testing, 254
   yeast overgrowth and, 76
Sugar-free products, 25
Sugary drinks, 23, 132
Sulforaphane, 98
Sulfur-containing amino acids, 52
Sunflower oil, 60
Sunshine, 70
Supercharged Hormone Diet
   detox phase
      forbidden foods, 60–61
      permitted foods, 62–63
      plan overview, 58–59
      reactions to, 63

week 1 meal plan, 233–41, 240–41
week 2 meal plan, 242–49, 250–51
Glyci-Med approach
  food guidelines, 88–89, 91–92, 171
  meal plans, 263–69, 270–71
  overview, 87–88, 262–63
  timing of meals/snacks in, 90–91
goal-setting checklist, 46–47
overview, 78
supplement plan, 67–70
transition week meal plan, 253–61
Supplements. *See also* Treatment
      Pyramid
  cautions regarding, 186, 188
  digestive enzymes, 72, 74
  fiber, 66
  hydrochloric acid, 74
  for improved sleep, 162–63
  for stress management, 161–62
Sushi, 93
Sweating, 168
Sweeteners
  in detox plan, 60–61, 63, 240–41,
      250–51
  in Glyci-Med approach, 91
  shopping tips, 118, 129
Sweet potatoes, 60

T₃/T₄. *See* Thyroid hormones
Tamari, 122
Taurine, 52, 197
Tea, 99, 133, 189–90, 204, 278
TEF (Thermic Effect of Food), 58 59
Television watching, 56
Tempeh, 134, 276
Testosterone
  foods/habits affecting, 209–10
  in food supply, 34
  hormonal health profile, 182–83
  low, 9, 30
  muscle growth effects, 13
  precursors, 202
  sleep quality and, 57
  supplement recommendations,
      208–10
  testing of, 224
Tests. *See* Benchmarking tests
Theanine, 99, 190
Thermic Effect of Food (TEF), 58–59
Thirst, 105
Thyme, 109

Thyroid hormones
  benefits, 211
  cortisol and, 198
  diet and, 32, 59, 63, 154, 212
  environmental toxins and, 30
  hormonal health profile, 184
  imbalance in, 9–10
  metabolism effects, 12, 81
  stress effects, 161
  supplement recommendations, 211–13
  testing of, 225–26
Tofu, 276
Tomato sauce, 124
Toxins, sources of, 29–31, 64–65. *See also*
      Detoxification
Tracking
  benchmarking tests
    list of, 226–28
    overview, 217–18
    test descriptions, 218–26
  Best Body Assessment, 39–49
  of weight, 160, 330, 331
  wellness tracker sheets, 329–30,
      332–59
Trans fats, 64, 91
Treatment Pyramid
  overview, 186–88, 187
  supplement recommendations
    inflammation, 188–90
    metabolism, 211–13
    mood hormones, 190–98
    renewal, 213–14
    sex hormones, 203–11
    strength, 214–16
    stress/anti-stress, 198–203
Treats, shopping tips, 129–30
Tribulus terrestris, 209
Triglycerides, testing of, 220
Triphala, 69
Tryptophan, 103, 106, 110, 163, 195
TSH (thyroid-stimulating hormone),
      9–10, 211, 225–26
Tuna, 133, 135
Turkey, 133–34, 155
Turmeric, 69, 109–10, 188–89, 204, 218
25-Hydroxy vitamin D₃, 226
Type 2 diabetes, 6
Tyrosine, 155–56, 212

Ulcers, 27, 72
Uric acid, testing of, 221

RECIPE INDEX